M000013024

MAKING
MEDICINE

MAKING
MONEY

MAKING MEDICINE

MAKING MONEY

DONALD DRAKE
and
MARIAN UHLMAN

of The Philadelphia Inquirer

Andrews and McMeel
A Universal Press Syndicate Company
Kansas City

Making Medicine, Making Money copyright © 1993 by Donald Drake and Marian Uhlman. All rights reserved. Printed in the United States of America. No part of this book may be used or reproduced in any manner whatsoever without written permission except in the case of reprints in the context of reviews. For information write Andrews and McMeel, a Universal Press Syndicate Company, 4900 Main Street, Kansas City, Missouri 64112.

Designed by Barrie Maguire

Library of Congress Cataloging-in-Publication Data

Drake, Donald, 1935–
    Making medicine, making money / Donald Drake and Marian Uhlman.
        p. cm.
    ISBN: 0-8362-8023-7: $5.95
        1. Pharmaceutical industry—United States. 2. Drugs—Prices-
-United States. 3. Prescription pricing—United States.
    I. Uhlman, Marian. II. Title.
    HD9666.5.D7   1993   93-12506
    338.4'76151'0973—dc20   CIP

First Printing, March 1993
Second Printing, March 1993

ATTENTION: SCHOOLS AND BUSINESSES

Andrews and McMeel books are available at quantity discounts with bulk purchase for educational, business, or sales promotional use. For information, please write to:
Special Sales Department, Andrews and McMeel,
4900 Main Street, Kansas City, Missouri 64112.

Contents

Acknowledgments

Making Medicine, Making Money first appeared as a five-part series in *The Philadelphia Inquirer.* That kind of series reaches print only in a newspaper with a deep commitment to telling a complicated story the way it needs to be told.

The commitment starts with an environment in which the staff is encouraged to do its best work and gets the freedom, time, and resources to do it. It's reinforced by editors who find ways to make ideas work rather than reasons why they cannot. And it continues with the generous allocation of space in the newspaper.

We're thankful we work for that kind of newspaper at a time when many other papers are turning to shorter, simpler stories in the mistaken belief that it's the only way to attract an audience nurtured on the thin diet of television. We are thankful, too, to *Inquirer* Editor Maxwell E.P. King, who is willing to fight for this kind of journalism, just as we are to his predecessor, Gene Roberts, who more than twenty years ago set the standards that we at the *Inquirer* now try to meet.

So many people helped us with *Making Medicine, Making Money* that it is difficult to remember everyone who should be included. But surely one name that must appear at the top is that of Assistant Managing Editor Lois Wark. She's a gifted, tenacious, tireless editor who weathered rewrite after rewrite and helped us bring to a conclusion what was turning into a difficult investigation of increasingly complicated data.

Likewise, we must acknowledge the contribution of Executive Editor Jim Naughton, whose critical eye encouraged us to make subtle changes that significantly improved the story, and Managing Editor Steve Lovelady, who rightfully takes pride in the art of minimalist editing that makes a major difference.

Long before the finished story was delivered to these editors, many people contributed their talents. Photographer Akira Suwa's enthusiasm, artistry, and curiosity added extra dimensions to our work. The project's graphic artist, Barbara F. Binik, brought life to numbers. And Al Hasbrouck used his incredible knowledge of computers to help us analyze data.

Marsha Canfield copy-edited the series, and Bob Filarsky designed the pages. Business Editor Jan Schaffer provided important insights, while our colleagues in the business-news department picked up the slack on daily news coverage so we could focus on the series.

Our research progressed more smoothly because of the research help of Denise Boal, an *Inquirer* librarian whose diligence and never-ending good humor were always appreciated.

John Duchneskie, a research assistant in the *Inquirer's* business-news department, was a stalwart friend who spent hours working with financial data and digging up information whenever we needed it.

We also wish to mention several colleagues who graciously shared their expertise about the business world: Don Barlett and Jim Steele, the *Inquirer's* well-regarded investigative reporting team; Craig Stock, the paper's business columnist; and Neill Borowski, the regional economics reporter.

We must also recognize the countless people who spent time with us, giving us the background to prepare the series. It's impossible to estimate how many people we interviewed here and abroad as we compiled the material.

Now that the articles have been turned into this book, more people helped shepherd it into print, many of them staffers with Andrews and McMeel. Our liaison with the publisher was Ken Bookman, director of the paper's New Ventures department, and to him, too, we owe a debt of thanks for his attention to detail. And Barrie Maguire's imagination came up with an engaging book design.

Finally, we thank our families, who ate many dinners without us, put up with our distractions when we were home, and encouraged us always.

DONALD DRAKE
MARIAN UHLMAN

Prologue

Prescription drug prices rose three times faster than inflation in the decade between 1981 and 1991, making the pharmaceutical industry the nation's most profitable business. Prescription drugs even exceeded the rapidly rising inflation rate for all other medical services. They now represent at least 10 percent of all medical costs in the United States.

While all Americans are feeling the crunch of higher prices, the burden has fallen most heavily on the elderly, who need medication more than others but who are less likely than working people to have prescription-drug insurance coverage. Pharmacy bills of $150 a month or more are not uncommon for people with multiple chronic conditions like heart disease and high blood pressure.

Why have pharmaceutical prices skyrocketed? And why hasn't the government taken action to assure Americans of access to needed medicines at reasonable prices? These are among the questions examined in this book.

The pharmaceutical industry, which made record profits in the 1980s, is facing unparalleled scrutiny as the issue of health care cost-containment takes center stage in Washington. The likelihood of price constraints being imposed on the drug industry has grown with the prospect that the United States will adopt some form of federally guaranteed health insurance.

Providing universal health coverage, while containing the soaring cost of medical care, are among the Clinton administration's greatest challenges. During the 1992 presidential campaign, Bill Clinton vowed to make health care reform a top priority of his administration. While the fight over how to do it is expected to be long and fierce, Clinton has insisted that legislation must contain at least two elements: cost controls and coverage for the 37 million Americans now without health insurance.

"If I could wave a magic wand tomorrow and do one thing for this economy, I would bring health costs in line with inflation and provide a basic [insurance] package to everybody," Clinton told students at a community college in Washington on December 7, 1992.

"We can't do anything else on the deficit if we fail to curtail the monster of spiraling health care costs," he said a week later, at the close of his economic conference in Little Rock on December 15.

Health care eats up about $800 billion, or 14 percent, of the nation's economic output, up from 6 percent in 1965. And prescription drugs are a part of that. Clinton is on record as favoring legislation that would restrict certain tax breaks of pharmaceutical companies that raised drug prices faster than the rate of inflation, as measured by the Consumer Price Index. Such legislation, aimed at tax breaks given to drug companies establishing plants in Puerto Rico, has been proposed by Sen. David Pryor (D., Ark.). Passage of any national health plan that does not contain effective cost-containment measures would only lead to greater drug price inflation, many experts say.

History has demonstrated the hazards of providing unlimited drug coverage. When the Japanese enacted their national health plan in 1961, drug sales increased so much that by the late 1980s they accounted for more than 30 percent of Japanese health expenditures, three times the American ratio. The Japanese government now is trying to bring down drug prices.

Some government officials and U.S. economists contend the proliferation of medical insurance plans that cover prescription drugs likewise has helped push up drug costs here. With someone other than the patient paying the bill, there is less concern about holding down prices.

Although it is the drug companies that set the high prices, they are not the only causes of the situation. Doctors have passively watched prices go up, handing out prescriptions for expensive drugs while accepting professional support—and sometimes favors—from the drug industry. Insurance companies have done little to use their huge buying power to force lower prices. Consumers have stoically accepted high prices without protest. It wasn't until AIDS activists started to demonstrate against the high cost of the AIDS drug AZT that citizens realized something could be done.

Most conspicuous by its inactivity has been the U.S. government and the Food and Drug Administration, whose lengthy approval process chews up the time available for companies to earn back their research and development costs while a drug is under patent and protected from competition. So the companies pass on the cost of these delays in the form of higher prices.

Some of that passivity may be coming to an end. "Drug company executives better not take any vacations" at the outset of the new administration, Senator Pryor, chairman of the Senate Special Committee on Aging, warned during the presidential campaign. "I want to pass something that contains drug price-inflation protection for all purchasers. And if that doesn't work, we're going to have to teach the industry that God doesn't grant patents, government does."

1.
Why are drug prices so high?

Eva Smalls Rozier has diabetes, a stomach ailment, and high blood pressure. To keep these problems in check, she takes prescription drugs costing $150 a month—more than she spends for food or her mortgage.

Transplant patient Joseph Pearlstein takes pills to keep his new heart from being rejected. The cost: $50 a day.

When John Forrest, Jr., suffered a heart attack, emergency room doctors shut off the attack with a drug that dissolved the blood clot causing it. The treatment cost $2,200.

Mary Nathan has a potentially lethal ailment called Gaucher's disease, which weakens bones and causes painful swelling of the spleen. Her drug costs $270,000 a year.

These patients have a variety of medical problems, from the ordinary to the unusual, but they have two things in common: They all owe their lives to drugs. And they are all captives of the $55 billion-a-year pharmaceutical industry.

It is the most profitable business in America.

It doesn't matter if the economy is flourishing or stagnating, if the jobless ranks have swelled or shrunk, if the inflation rate is high or low, or even if America is at war or at peace. The pharmaceutical industry rakes in the cash. No other legal business consistently makes as large a profit.

Drawing on scientific breakthroughs in government, academic, and commercial laboratories in the last two decades, pharmaceutical companies have turned out one wonder drug after another—drugs that reduce cholesterol, protect organ transplants from rejection, heal ulcers, shrink prostate glands, ease depression, even drugs that shut off heart attacks.

Wonderful drugs—if you can afford them. A growing number of Americans cannot. The prices are just too high.

Prescription drug prices rose three times faster than inflation in the last decade, and the industry has circumvented every effort by the government to contain prices. Drug companies increase prices without fear, protected from competition by patents that give them monopolies on their chemical compounds. Even when patents expire and generic competition moves in, prices don't go down—they go up. The major companies simply charge more for their brand-name drugs to make up for their lost share of the market, knowing that brand-name loyalty will keep doctors prescribing their drugs, despite higher prices.

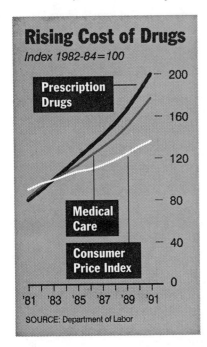

Rising Cost of Drugs
Index 1982-84=100

Prescription Drugs

Medical Care

Consumer Price Index

200 160 120 80 40 0

'81 '83 '85 '87 '89 '91

SOURCE: Department of Labor

This loyalty is created by spending billions of dollars a year courting doctors—more money is spent on sales representatives and promotion than on research and development.

In the world of prescription drugs, the normal rules of the marketplace don't apply. Here, the person who pays for the product—the patient—isn't the one who selects it. And the drug consumer, confronting pain, illness, or death, doesn't have the option of doing without.

Drug company executives defend their prices by citing the high cost and risky nature of pharmaceutical research and development. But a close examination of the industry shows that it avoids risk in many ways.

The companies make "me-too" drugs that duplicate already-proven successes. They stand back while smaller companies and university scientists do the lengthy and costly basic research, and then step in when it looks as if a potentially profitable drug is at hand. They focus their research on the search for blockbuster drugs, to the detriment of other potential treatments.

Drug companies benefit substantially from government and academic research and then turn around and slap premium prices on drugs developed at taxpayer expense. The National Cancer Institute, for example, and the scientists it funds have played an important role in developing some seventy cancer drugs. Still, cancer drugs are among the most expensive on the market.

Wyeth-Ayerst Laboratories did virtually none of the R&D on Norplant, which was supported by government and philanthropic money. But Wyeth-Ayerst is selling the long-acting contraceptive in this country for almost four times the price charged in Europe by the company that manufactures it.

This may come as a shock, but it shouldn't. Americans routinely pay more for drugs than anyone else in the world.

By the three most important measures of profitability—return on equity, return on sales, and return on assets—the drug industry has ranked at or near the top year after year after year.

In 1991, while the rest of American industry was experiencing a sharp decline in profits, many brand-name pharmaceutical companies were posting earnings 15 percent to 20 percent over the previous year.

Among the *Fortune* 500 drug companies, the median return on equity was 26 percent—that is, every dollar invested was making twenty-six cents profit. That was twice the median for all *Fortune* 500 industries. And the largest American drug firm, Merck & Co., was making forty-three cents on every dollar. Pharmaceuticals were doing twenty-six times better than autos, three times better than oil, and two times better than publishing.

It's not just the big *Fortune* 500 drug companies that are so profitable. Even when smaller companies with smaller profits are considered, the drug industry comes out on top.

The *Philadelphia Inquirer* asked Value Line, an investment advisory service, to compile data on industry performance over a twenty-year period. The sample of nineteen drug companies contained a mixture of large and small firms, biotechnology companies, and generic firms.

An *Inquirer* analysis of the Value Line data showed that for:

- Return on equity, the drug industry finished first among eighty-seven industries, followed by soft drinks and toiletries.
- Return on assets, pharmaceuticals led eighty-six industries.
- Return on sales, the drug industry ranked third, behind two electric utility groups.

The most profitable industry, by any measure: *Fortune* 500 . . .

Performance of six selected industries:

- Drug industry
- Computer & office equipment
- Motor vehicles & parts
- Food
- Petroleum refining
- Publishing, printing

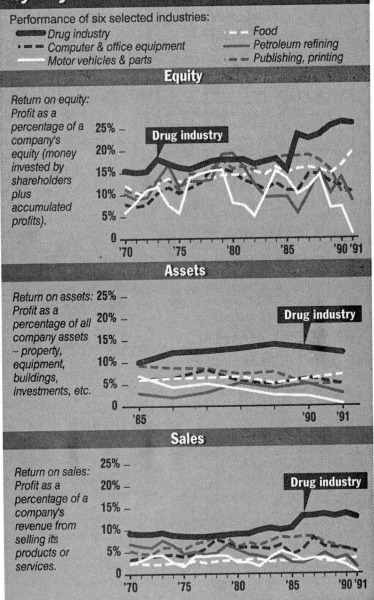

Equity

Return on equity: Profit as a percentage of a company's equity (money invested by shareholders plus accumulated profits).

Drug industry

25% – 20% – 15% – 10% – 5% – 0

'70   '75   '80   '85   '90 '91

Assets

Return on assets: Profit as a percentage of all company assets – property, equipment, buildings, investments, etc.

Drug industry

25% – 20% – 15% – 10% – 5% – 0

'85   '90   '91

Sales

Return on sales: Profit as a percentage of a company's revenue from selling its products or services.

Drug industry

25% – 20% – 15% – 10% – 5% – 0

'70   '75   '80   '85   '90 '91

SOURCES: *Fortune* magazine, Value Line Institutional Services

6

... and a Value Line sampling of large and small companies.

Performance of six selected industries:
- Drug industry
- Computer & peripherals
- Auto & truck
- Food processing
- Petro-integrated
- Newspapers

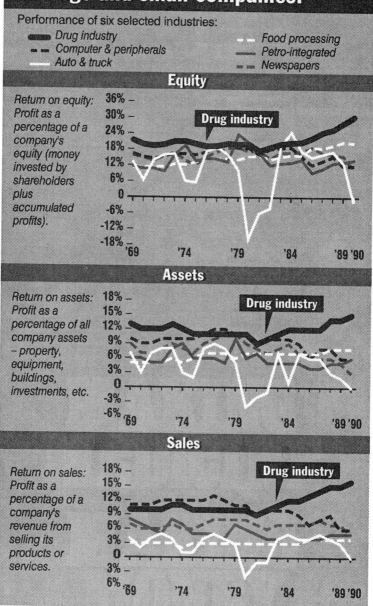

Equity

Return on equity: Profit as a percentage of a company's equity (money invested by shareholders plus accumulated profits).

36% – 30% – 24% – 18% – 12% – 6% – 0 -6% – -12% – -18% –

Drug industry

'69 '74 '79 '84 '89 '90

Assets

Return on assets: Profit as a percentage of all company assets – property, equipment, buildings, investments, etc.

18% – 15% – 12% – 9% – 6% – 3% – 0 -3% – -6%

Drug industry

'69 '74 '79 '84 '89 '90

Sales

Return on sales: Profit as a percentage of a company's revenue from selling its products or services.

18% – 15% – 12% – 9% – 6% – 3% – 0 3% – 6%

Drug industry

'69 '74 '79 '84 '89 '90

The Philadelphia Inquirer / B.F. BINIK

As for the industry's performance over twenty years, the Value Line data showed it became much more profitable during the 1980s, a time when companies were aggressively raising prices.

Prescription drug prices have shot up 147 percent in the last decade, a period during which prices overall rose 50 percent. The effect of higher prices is being felt by all Americans, but particularly hard hit are many older people on Medicare, which doesn't cover prescription drugs outside a hospital. It is not uncommon for a single pill to cost $1.50 or $2, and people with multiple chronic conditions must take three or more pills a day for the rest of their lives. That means pharmacy bills of $150 a month or more.

Retirees on fixed incomes have watched in alarm as drug prices climbed two to three times faster than the cost-of-living adjustments in their Social Security checks. Prescription drugs are a bigger out-of-pocket expense for them than doctors or hospitals. Many older Americans are going without drugs that could relieve their pain, control their disease, or even save their lives. Many others try to stretch out their prescriptions by taking less than the effective doses.

Workers are feeling the pinch, too. With health care costs soaring, more and more companies are seeking ways to reduce expensive employee benefits, such as prescription drug plans. More than half of all out-patient prescription costs—for young and old alike—are paid by the buyer, not by insurance.

Many middle-class families are turning to public health clinics for vaccinations, which can cost $150 for a child's first two years.

Drugs represent at least 10 percent of all medical costs, according to Stephen Schondelmeyer, a leading economist on the drug industry.

Americans paid an average of 54 percent more for the exact same drugs sold in Europe, according to a 1989 international comparison by the Belgian Consumer Association, a research group. And prices charged by manufacturers are 32 percent higher, on average, in the United States than in Canada, according to a 1992 study by the General Accounting Office, a congressional agency.

The United States is one of very few industrialized nations that do not control drug prices. Other countries, which operate national health care systems, hold down prices rather than passing them on to their voters in the form of higher taxes.

Because the U.S. government does not try to control pharmaceutical prices in any systematic way, and because the United States is the industry's largest single market, many drug companies—foreign and U.S. alike—look to this country for their biggest profits.

Because drug manufacturers attribute the high U.S. prices to the need to maintain large research-and-development budgets, and because the United States represents about 30 percent of worldwide sales, American consumers are supporting much of the R&D costs for the world.

Members of Congress have become concerned. And with a new president who says he is committed to addressing the issue of runaway health care costs, the question is sure to get louder:

Why are drug prices so high?

They sat at a green table before TV cameras and congressmen, and each of the witnesses had a horror story to tell the scores of people who had packed the third-floor Senate hearing room.

They were testifying at a hearing on January 21, 1992, on the Orphan Drug Act, a federal law that encourages drug firms to develop medicines for uncommon diseases by giving them a seven-year monopoly on those drugs.

The witnesses, several the victims of chronic and debilitating medical problems, were pleading for changes in the law to make it possible for cheaper, generic drugs to reach the market.

The Tom Hires family of Paola, Kans., talked about their fourteen-year-old son and told the senators how his growth had been retarded by radiation treatments for a brain tumor. The growth hormones they were giving him were helping, they said, but the drug cost $3,300 a month.

Cindy Smith from Salt Lake City, Utah, bent toward the microphone and told the saga of her two-and-a-half-year-old son, Justin, who has the physique of a six-month-old baby. He, too, was getting the costly growth hormone.

"We're doing everything we can to pay our share of the cost of hormone treatments and other medical expenses," said Smith, who tried to hold back tears. "Our whole life is devoted to paying medical bills. We can't afford to do more."

Derek Hodel, the executive director for People with AIDS Health Group, asked the senators to change the law so that competing firms could make a drug that helps AIDS patients combat a severe form of pneumonia. The manufacturer of the drug, protected from competition by the Orphan Drug Act, had increased its price by 400 percent in just three years in the 1980s, Hodel said.

Sitting in a wheelchair, Mary Nathan of Silver Spring, Md., told the senators that she had Gaucher's disease, a hereditary illness that weakens bones, enlarges the spleen and liver, saps energy, and threatens death. The new medicine Ceredase was keeping her alive, at a cost of $270,000 a year. The thirty-seven-year-old woman said she worried about what will happen to her once she reaches the maximum amount that her insurance will pay.

Finally, Herb Jacobson of Denver explained how his daughter, who also has Gaucher's disease, refuses to take the medicine because it would use up all of the lifetime benefits of her family's health plan. "These Gaucher patients have been transformed into victims," Jacobson said, his voice revealing passion and even greater frustration. "They are being victimized, assaulted by the deadliest weapons in this era: Unbridled greed."

The drug industry says it is a very competitive business.

"I think the industry itself is sort of a free-enterprise, liberal economist's dream," Gerald J. Mossinghoff, president of the Pharmaceutical Manufacturers Association, the industry's trade group and lobbying arm, said in 1989 before a Senate subcommittee looking into high drug prices.

The trade association likes to cite the ulcer medicine, Tagamet, as an example of the marketplace at work. Actually, it's a better example of drug companies at work, carefully avoiding price competition.

Tagamet was introduced in the United States in 1977 by SmithKline Corp. (now SmithKline Beecham). For six years, SmithKline had a lock on the ulcer market. No other drug even came close to matching Tagamet's effectiveness.

Then in 1983, Glaxo Pharmaceuticals introduced an equally good drug, Zantac. Glaxo charged a premium for the drug, claiming that it had fewer side effects. This was followed by two more anti-ulcer drugs that worked on the same biologic principle—Merck & Co.'s Pepcid, introduced in 1986, and Eli Lilly & Co.'s Axid, approved for marketing in 1988. "Now this is a market economy well at work," Mossinghoff told the subcomittee.

What he didn't explain was how the companies responded to this competition.

SmithKline didn't cut the price of Tagamet when Zantac entered the market. Instead, it held the price steady for one year, suggesting that SmithKline was waiting and watching what Zantac would do. Then the prices of both drugs moved upward in parallel fashion.

With two major ulcer drugs already on the market, the normal expectation would be that Lilly and Merck would try to undersell Glaxo and SmithKline. But they came in a little higher than Tagamet. And neither company has lowered its price since.

The companies simply did not compete on price.

Zantac is the biggest-selling drug in the history of the pharmaceutical industry. In 1991, sales topped $3 billion. And Tagamet? It's number thirteen in sales, at just over $1 billion a year.

As evidence of its competitiveness, the industry provides these figures: Three-fourths of industry sales are by the twenty largest companies, and no single company controls more than 7.6 percent of the market.

But the companies don't really compete with one another, across a broad market. They dominate different segments of the market where their patents, and their strengths, have been developed. In these specialized markets, any one company's presence can be 50 percent or more.

Take, for example, the most popular class of anticholesterol drugs. Two of the three brands are made by Merck, which launched its revolutionary drug, Mevacor, in 1987. In 1991, Merck introduced a second drug in this class, Zocor, and asked a competitor, SmithKline Beecham, to help sell it. By combining the sales forces of the two companies, Merck was able to continue dominating the cholesterol drug market, while sharing the profits with SmithKline.

Instead of competing on price, brand-name companies in the United States compete on developing patentable products, said Peter Temin, a professor at the Massachusetts Institute of Technology and a historian on the industry. That is because patent laws give drug companies near monopolies in the treatment of specific medical problems.

The patent law is immensely valuable to drug companies.

"Patents are not terribly significant in other industries—not to the extent they are in the drug industry, where you have a virtual monopoly," said Christina Heuer, a financial analyst with Smith Barney, Harris Upham & Co. in New York. Patents are "not only an ironclad barrier to competition," but they provide protection against "anybody scooping your discovery during the long product-development period," she said.

Patents are granted for seventeen years and can be extended up to five years to make up for time a drug is under Food and Drug Administration review. It can take up to twelve years to move a potential medicine from test tube through human drug trials and past regulatory review, the industry says. Thus a drug's commercial life under patent protection is usually between seven and ten years.

Heuer said that she could think of no other industry that has the

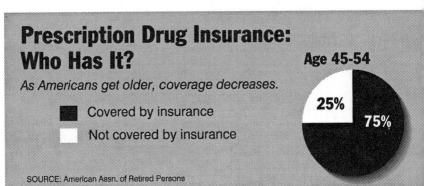

Prescription Drug Insurance: Who Has It?

Age 45-54

As Americans get older, coverage decreases.

■ Covered by insurance

□ Not covered by insurance

25%

75%

SOURCE: American Assn. of Retired Persons

"monolithic patent protection" that the pharmaceutical industry has. "That is the cause of their uniquely high profit margins," she said.

When industry executives talk about profits, they sometimes contradict themselves. "They are torn," said MIT professor Stewart Myers. "They want to tell the politicians they are not exceptionally profitable, and they want to tell securities analysts they are."

When talking to reporters, Pharmaceutical Manufacturers Association officials say comparisons with other industries, such as the *Fortune* 500 companies, exaggerate the drug industry's profits. Instead, they say the drug industry's profitability should be compared to other companies with comparable research-and-development spending. Even when that was done in a recent government study, the drug industry was consistently more profitable.

The people who led the companies to these profits are rewarded handsomely. The average compensation in 1991 for the chief executive officers of the eight biggest American pharmaceutical companies was in excess of $5 million.

Richard D. Wood, who retired as chief executive officer of Eli Lilly & Co. in 1991, received $10.11 million in 1991 ($2.21 million in salary and bonuses and $7.89 million in stock), making him the twelfth-best-paid executive in the United States, according to a *Fortune* survey.

Number thirteen was P. Roy Vagelos, chairman and chief executive officer of Merck & Co., who received $9.70 million.

Wood's compensation was two and a half times more than that of Campbell Soup Co. president David Johnson, fifty times more than that of the president of the United States, and about 250 times more than the median income of a family of four.

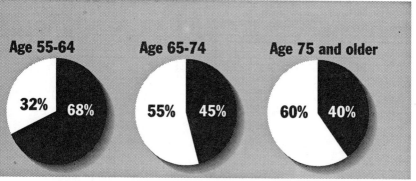

The Philadelphia Inquirer / B.F. BINIK

Eva Smalls Rozier, 48, couldn't keep paying $150 for the drugs that kept her alive.

Prescription drugs to control her diabetes, high blood pressure, and stomach problems were the single biggest item in her budget, surpassing the $30 she spent each week on food and the $99 she spent each month on the mortgage for her home in West Philadelphia.

For more than a year, ever since she lost her job typing data into a computer because of her poor vision, Rozier had been buying the drugs with money taken from her savings. The savings were fast disappearing. So she decided to take a chance. She stopped taking her medicine.

One month later, Rozier was wheeled into the intensive-care unit of the University of Pennsylvania Medical Center, near death from malignant hypertension, a lethal complication of uncontrolled high blood pressure.

When she was released from the hospital ten days later, doctors and nurses warned Rozier that she had no choice: She had to take the drugs. A hospital social worker advised her to spend her savings so she would qualify for Medicaid. That's what she did.

"We are not an unprofitable industry," said Mossinghoff of the Pharmaceutical Manufacturers Association.

Mossinghoff says that it is reasonable for drug companies to be well compensated for all the work that companies do to bring that bottle of pills to the bedside. "The fact is that something of enormous value goes into those tiny tablets," Mossinghoff said at the association's 1992 annual meeting. "We can quantify that value by looking at drug development costs."

The trade group estimates that it costs $231 million to bring one successful drug to market. That factors in the costs of other drugs under development that don't make it. The costs have grown from $54 million in 1976, Mossinghoff said.

Any cutback in financial resources "would inevitably lead to a cutback in research-and-development expenditures," Mossinghoff said in an interview. "And that would inevitably lead to less good medicine being produced by our companies."

He pointed to France and Canada, both of which have price controls. "They're not as innovative as they used to be. If the United States goes into that mode, you have got big problems—you've got Alzheimer's with you for a long time."

"It is very expensive to come up with new products," said Fred Hassan, president of Wyeth-Ayerst Laboratories in St. Davids, Pa. "We are trying to do that every year. It is extremely risky. It is absolutely critical, the free-market principle of pricing. If you discourage initiative, why should people [investors] take the risk?"

Drug executives define that risk as a 1-in-5,000 chance. Those are the odds, they say, that any compound identified in their laboratories will end up on the market. Even among those drugs that make it, only three out of ten recoup their research and development costs, they say.

There is a difference, however, between financial risk and the R&D risks that the industry repeatedly cites. It is true that any given research project entails considerable risk, with the likelihood of failure far outweighing the likelihood of success. But the overall strategy of a company, including the research effort, is designed in such a way that the risks to investors are kept to a minimum.

For example, many big companies spread their research risk by developing variations of successful drugs already on the market—so-called me-too drugs. That is less of a gamble than trying to find a breakthrough drug—a major advance in treatment.

Most companies won't get involved in a research project if they don't think it will pay off in ten years, industry researchers say.

Some drug company executives, including Hassan of Wyeth-Ayerst, cite the many mergers in the industry as evidence of how risky the business is. Since 1985, SmithKline Beckman Corp. of Philadelphia has merged with Beecham Group, a British company; Bristol-Meyers Co. of New York bought Squibb Corp. of Princeton, N.J.; Rorer Group of Fort Washington, Pa., aligned itself with the drug operations of Rhone-Poulenc of France. American Home Products Corp. of New York, the parent of Wyeth-Ayerst, itself took part in a major merger when it acquired A.H. Robins.

"If you do not innovate in this industry . . . you will be forced to merge," said Fred Telling, vice president, planning and policy, for U.S. Pharmaceuticals Group of Pfizer Inc. But even mergers are an effective way of minimizing risk to investors when a pharmaceutical company has consistently failed to make important research discoveries.

A classic example is SmithKline Beckman. Investors became acutely aware in mid-1988 that the Philadelphia firm could not sustain its profit growth. Sales from its biggest-selling drugs—Tagamet for ulcers and Dyazide for hypertension—had dropped, and the company didn't have any new blockbuster drugs ready for the market.

Even though SmithKline was far from unprofitable, the company announced in April 1989 that it would merge with Beecham. Since then, the value of the company's stock has nearly doubled.

"From a financial, economic point of view, the mergers help to improve the risk profile" of a company, said Kurt Landgraff, executive vice president of the Du Pont Merck Pharmaceutical Co.

Like many businesses in the 1980s, drug companies arranged mergers for a variety of reasons: to gain in size, to pick up product lines, to show profit growth, or to strengthen their position in the global marketplace. Of the ten large American drug companies involved in mergers since 1985, only one, A.H. Robins, was a failing company. It filed for bankruptcy in 1985, as lawsuits mounted over its Dalkon Shield intrauterine birth-control device.

Here's what Richard M. Furlaud, chairman and CEO of Squibb, said after the 1989 announcement of its partnership with Bristol-Myers: "This is a merger of two very strong companies. We certainly could have kept going on our own. This is a combination of two strengths."

And Robert Cawthorn, chairman and CEO of Rorer Group of Fort Washington, Pa., in 1990, about teaming up with Rhone-Poulenc: "In my view, the time to do something innovative like this is when things are going well, not badly. That's exactly the situation we are in. That's exactly why we put together a transaction which I believe is great for our shareholders."

At worst, mergers by drug companies represent "a failure to manage risk," said Samuel Isaly, a New York financial analyst. Yet individual failures do not mean that the industry itself is risky, he said.

In other words, those three out of ten drugs that hit the jackpot more than just pay for the other seven on the market and the thousands that didn't make it—they provide big profits, as well.

That is why financial analysts rate the stocks of major pharmaceutical companies as slightly less risky than the stock market as a whole.

It's why there are no more bankruptcies among drug companies than among other American businesses.

It is why most drug companies increase their sales and profits year after year after year.

It is why drug stocks have climbed in value almost three times more than the Standard & Poor's average for five hundred leading companies since 1980.

It is why the federal Office of Technology Assessment recently wrote that the financial returns of drug companies "were higher than was required to reward investors for the time and risks incurred."

And that is why the pharmaceutical industry consistently is the most profitable industry in America.

Every morning, heart transplant patient Joseph Pearlstein begins his day by sitting down at his kitchen table in northeast Philadelphia and counting out the pills he must take to stay alive.

He counts out round pills and rectangular pills and triangular pills and oval pills. Before he is through, the thirty-nine-year-old biomedical technician will have counted out 35½ pills (on even-numbered days, 31½), not including the multivitamins, calcium supplement, and occasional Tylenol he also takes.

Pearlstein is a pharmaceutical company's dream come true and an insurance company's nightmare. He's a classic example of the extraordinary things that modern drugs can do and the extraordinary expense of doing them.

Without the pills, Pearlstein couldn't live more than a few months before his transplanted heart was rejected or he died of other medical complications. So each morning he counts out his pills, knowing that it will probably be the most important thing he will do that day.

To prevent his heart from being rejected in an immunologic reaction, each day he must take six cyclosporin pills, which cost a total of $27.96; two-and-a-half Imuran ($2.52); and five prednisone ($1.30). To counteract the hypertension and fluid retention caused by the prednisone, he takes two Vasotec ($2.85) and two Lasix (40 cents). To counteract the gastric intestinal distress and prevent ulcers that could be caused by all the drugs, he takes two Zantac ($4.48).

Pearlstein also must take pills for toxoplasmosis, a parasitic infection he developed because the antirejection drugs had reduced his immunity. To treat it, he takes four sulfadiazine (84 cents), two Leucovorin ($6), one Daraprim (67 cents), and one Trimethoprim (51 cents).

Taking all these chemical compounds makes him prone to migraines. For this he takes Pamelor ($1.39 a capsule). It also apparently increases his cholesterol levels. For this he takes six niacin (16 cents) and one Mevacor ($3).

He takes the full complement of pills every other day, for a total daily cost of $52.08. On alternate days he skips the Lasix, Daraprim, and Trimethoprim, reducing his daily cost to $50.50.

Because Pearlstein's drugs are periodically adjusted, it's difficult to say what his annual bill will be. But if nothing changed, it would be $18,721.64. Usually the drug bill for transplant patients goes down over time. Fortunately for Pearlstein, he is covered by insurance, which pays most of the cost.

Pearlstein uses so many drugs and drugs of such a specialized nature that he doesn't just go to the drugstore and buy them.

He orders them from Stadtlanders Pharmacy, a nationwide mail-order drug-supply house in Pittsburgh that specializes in patients requiring extensive medication.

Stadtlanders has more than 12,000 patients like Pearlstein.

Drug company executives don't talk much about how they arrive at the price of a drug.

"Pharmaceutical prices are hard to understand because people look at a tablet or a capsule and say, 'It can't be more than four or five cents worth of ingredient in there,'" said Robert C. Black, president of the U.S. pharmaceutical unit of ICI of Great Britain. "That's absolutely correct. Why should you sell it for sixty cents when there is only five cents of chemicals? It is to cover all the other ongoing costs. . . . That's hard for people to understand."

Time and again, government researchers have tried to find out.

The General Accounting Office ran into a wall of silence in 1992 when it undertook a study of drug-price inflation. The congressional agency's report said, "Companies' explanations for the drug-price increases were general and provided few details because they consider information on pricing decisions to be confidential and proprietary."

The Office of Technology Assessment also had to do without specific R&D costs in its preparation of a massive new study on pharmaceutical R&D. A draft of the agency's report said drug companies "have demonstrated a willingness to actively resist providing access to congressional agencies to this proprietary data."

So drug pricing is a mystery, said MIT's Temin. "The drug companies do not talk about it."

They don't have to. The U.S. Supreme Court has ruled that drug companies don't have to open their books, saying that most pricing

Top 15 Pharmaceutical Companies Worldwid

For the year ended Dec. 31, 1991.[1]

Rank	Company	Country
1	Glaxo Holdings Plc.	Britain
2	Merck & Co.	United States
3	Bristol-Myers Squibb Corp.	United States
4	Hoechst A.G.	Germany
5	Ciba-Geigy Ltd.	Switzerland
6	Sandoz Ltd.	Switzerland
7	SmithKline Beecham Plc.	Britain
8	Bayer A.G.	Germany
9	Roche Holdings Ltd.	Switzerland
10	Eli Lilly & Co.	United States
11	American Home Products Corp.	United States
12	Rhone-Poulenc Rorer Inc.	United States
13	Johnson & Johnson	United States
14	Pfizer Inc.	United States
15	Abbott Laboratories	United States

[1] Except Glaxo (June 1992) and Johnson & Johnson (January 1992).
[2] Dollar conversions are based on average annual exchange rates for 1991
[3] Percentage change in U.S. dollars over previous year.

SOURCES: Mehta & Isaly, Scrip's Pharmaceutical Company League Tables

information is proprietary. Most of the information the industry does give to explain its prices is general and incomplete, or open to challenge.

For instance, company spokespeople highlight how much of the sales dollar is spent on R&D (roughly 16 cents) but are much less forthcoming about how much is allocated to marketing.

One of the few breakdowns of drug costs by an independent researcher was done in 1989 by Stephen Schondelmeyer, the University of Minnesota economist who is an expert in the drug industry and a pharmacist. He now says that about 22 percent of a drug's cost goes for marketing and about 16 percent for R&D.

As for the $231 million research figure, it not only includes direct development costs but also the cost of money—money the investor could expect to earn elsewhere during the time it takes to develop a drug. That amounts to about $117 million—a little more than half the total.

For this $231 million figure, the Pharmaceutical Manufacturers Asso-

harmaceutical sales[2] (n billions)	% change from 1990[3]	Drugs as a % of sales	% of sales in U.S.
$7.247	+19.5%	100.0%	40%
$7.225	+13.5%	84.0%	45%
$5.908	+12.3%	52.9%	60%
$5.429	+8.8%	19.1%	10%
$4.611	+8.8%	31.4%	40%
$4.440	+8.6%	47.4%	30%
$4.370	+3.0%	52.7%	40%
$4.309	+9.7%	16.9%	30%
$4.119	+19.1%	51.6%	35%
$4.031	+8.8%	70.4%	70%
$4.018	+16.0%	56.8%	60%
$3.824	+31.1%	100.0%	25%
$3.795	+14.9%	30.5%	40%
$3.770	+16.6%	54.3%	40%
$3.512	+11.1%	51.1%	50%

The Philadelphia Inquirer / B.F. BINIK

ciation cites a study by Tufts University's Center for the Study of Drug Development, which receives financial support from the industry. The company data behind this figure cannot be examined because the Tufts researchers say it was provided on a confidential basis.

"It is impossible for us to pull out the costs of the successful projects that contribute, directly or indirectly, to the discovery and development of the rare compound that eventually becomes a prescription medicine," P. Roy Vagelos, Merck's chairman, wrote in *Science* magazine in 1991.

"It is also impossible for us to isolate costs for all the individual projects that fail. What we do know is that, on an industry-wide basis, counting all the investments in the failed and successful projects, it costs $231 million, on average, to bring one new prescription medicine to market in the United States."

The drug industry has tried to calm the skeptics by saying that, whatever the price, prescription drugs are still the most cost-effective medical care going. They are cheap compared to the surgery they sometimes replace, executives say.

"I don't think we compete on price, we compete on value," said Black of ICI. "You price therapy based on the value it gives and what you need to recover in order to compensate for all the research and development that has gone into it. If the product has value and it is more expensive, it will be used. If it doesn't have value and it is more expensive, it won't be used. It is as simple as that."

What does the industry mean by value?

Isn't it better to spend $1,000 on hypertension medicines than to pay $41,000 for heart surgery? executives ask.

"You price value as perceived by the consumer," said Landgraff, of Du Pont Merck Pharmaceuticals.

"If they really appreciate the value, many patients would pay substantially more," said Fred Telling of Pfizer. "Medicines are undervalued. . . .The value to patients is far higher than the charge. Some people believe we make too much money. What's too much money? We are fundamentally in the business of innovation. The risks are there and known."

Vagelos of Merck, who declined to be interviewed, wrote in his *Science* article: "One of the most difficult challenges faced in marketing a new prescription medicine is the question of how much to charge for it. What is the value to society? To the individual patient? If cost effectiveness were the final arbiter of pricing decisions, most pharmaceutical prices could justifiably be much higher than they are."

If the value of a drug is comparable to the cost of surgery, or relief from pain and suffering, or even death, how do you put a price on that?

"You charge what the traffic will bear," said Heuer, the Smith Barney analyst. "It is clear in the pharmaceutical industry that drugs taken for a short period of time, like analgesics and antibiotics, are more expensive than heart and arthritis medicines. It is easier to get someone to pay a great deal for a drug that they will take for a week or a month, especially if they are dying. If it is a drug to extend their life, that is worth something."

John Forrest, Jr., never worried about the high cost of prescription drugs, at least not as far as he was concerned.

Robust, active, and apparently in perfect health, the thirty-eight-year-old Philadelphia electrician never took drugs, not even aspirin.

But that changed a little before midnight on May 19, when he suffered a heart attack.

Shortly after he arrived in the emergency room of a local hospital, doctors recommended TPA, a bioengineered drug that breaks up the blood clots that cause heart attacks. In severe pain and afraid he might die, Forrest agreed. The drug was administered at 1 A.M. At precisely 3:30 A.M., Forrest remembers, the pain stopped.

"The pain disappeared suddenly," Forrest said, recalling that night several months later. "It didn't gradually go away. It went away just like that," he said, snapping his fingers.

TPA was a miracle as far as Forrest was concerned. It had value. But the miracle was expensive.

The single infusion cost $2,200.

Most Americans don't think about the cost of prescription drugs until they walk into a drugstore, hand the druggist a prescription, and then, a few minutes later, get back a very little bottle and a very large bill. Because the encounter takes place in a drugstore, there's a tendency to blame the druggist.

The fact is that the cost of a prescription drug is determined primarily by the manufacturer. Sixty-nine cents of every sales dollar goes to the manufacturer, according to Schondelmeyer, who did a study for the federal Health Care Financing Administration in 1989 and recently updated the figures.

Until 1980, drug prices were increasing more slowly than the rate of inflation. But then something happened. Prices started climbing rapidly, increasing at twice the rate of other consumer prices. During the first half of the 1980s, drug prices went up 81 percent, compared with 48 percent for other items.

Mossinghoff, the Pharmaceutical Manufacturers Association's president, told Congress in 1985 that it was a "short-term" development, presumably something that would stabilize in a year or two.

But that's not what happened. In the next six years, prices soared another 66 percent, more than double the rate for other goods. If a worker's salary had increased at the same rate over the twelve years, a $36,000-a-year family would be bringing in an additional $442 a week, or $59,000 a year.

"What we were trying to do, quite honestly, is play a little bit of catch-up," said Black of ICI, based in Wilmington, Del. "I can't speak for other companies. We didn't have price increases for many, many years. We absorbed a lot of the inflationary costs. . . . We simply got to the point our margins were shrinking. We couldn't afford to do that."

Something else happened, too, said Joseph Scodari, vice president and general manager of U.S. pharmaceuticals at Rhone-Poulenc Rorer

Inc. in Collegeville, Pa. A sophisticated group of business managers joined the pharmaceutical industry, which had been focused more on research than on marketing. When they arrived, Scodari said, they recognized that "pharmaceutical prices were grossly underpriced. They took action to raise prices."

Schondelmeyer said the drug manufacturers were clearly the ones fueling the price increases.

The average prescription costs $22.50 today, compared to $6.62 in 1980, according to the National Association of Chain Drugstores.

Even so, the drug industry argues that drug prices are a minor part of health care inflation. Pharmaceutical Manufacturers Association officials say that drug costs constitute only about 4.5 percent of the nation's health dollar. They acknowledge that in-hospital and Health Maintenance Organization drugs and mail-order sales are not included in this figure. Including them, the figure comes to between 7 percent and 8 percent, industry officials say.

Schondelmeyer, however, says the real figure is more than 10 percent of total health costs, when all prices, including retail and not just manufacturers' prices, are tabulated.

The debate over drug prices has raged in one form or another for more than three decades. Senator Estes Kefauver of Tennessee launched an inquiry into the pricing practices of the pharmaceutical industry in the late 1950s and unearthed startling facts: The industry reported twice the rate of profit that other manufacturing firms in the United States were making. Americans paid much more for medicine than people in other countries. And much of the research duplicated medicines already on the market.

The drug industry's response: Pharmaceutical prices were a bargain compared to the value that drugs give. The high returns generated by successful medicines offset the high cost of the many unsuccessful attempts. And high profits were needed to maintain a healthy research pipeline.

A generation later, little has changed.

Every year, some time before Valentine's Day, Mary Ellen Sampson leaves her winter home in Yuma, Ariz., and makes a special shopping trip to the Mexican border town of Algodones. The goal of these trips is the ulcer medicine Tagamet.

She never makes the trips during the first days of the month because that's when American retirees receive their Social Security checks and travel down to Algodones to buy their prescription drugs at a fraction of the price in Yuma or elsewhere in the United States. On those days, the

California Pharmacy in Algodones is filled with American senior citizens, patiently waiting on long lines to beat the high cost of prescription drugs.

For fifty years, the Mexican government has set drug prices. Drug companies must apply for, and justify, any price increase. As a result, a bottle of pills that costs $10 in Mexico costs $20 to $40 in the United States.

Last winter, Sampson picked up four bottles of Tagamet, paying about $15 for a bottle of 100 pills, or roughly 70 percent less than in a U.S. pharmacy. When she got home, Sampson wrapped the bottles in white tissue paper with red hearts, and sent one off to each of her four ulcer-prone children in Maine, Montana, Washington, and California.

Trying to fend off the anger and criticism, drug company officials say they have moderated price increases. And they have.

In 1989, prices increased 9.1 percent.

In 1990, they increased 8.9 percent.

In 1991, the increase slowed to 8.3 percent.

And in the twelve months ended November 30, 1992, the price increase was 6.6 percent.

The industry cites these figures from the government's Producer Price Index, which measures increases in manufacturers' prices, as opposed to retail prices used for the Consumer Price Index. Comparable consumer figures are about one percentage point higher, reflecting the actual costs patients pay.

But there's another important comparison: While drug price increases have slowed, the economy has slowed even more. So in the period when drug prices as measured by the Producer Price Index rose 6.6 percent, all manufacturers' prices rose an average 1.1 percent. In other words, drug companies were raising their prices six times faster than other manufacturers.

"We are under attack as never before," Paul Freiman, chief executive officer of Syntex Corp. and chairman of the Pharmaceutical Manufacturers Association, told the trade group's annual meeting in May 1992. "And I feel unless we can strengthen the industry's immune system, we will be under constant and even more severe attack that could well affect our viability to research, develop, and bring to the market the world's best medicines."

Seven companies have announced that they would keep their price increases within the rate of general inflation.

"We are trying to balance social responsibility with responsibility toward our shareholders," said Black, whose firm is one of those committed to restraining price increases. "And that's a fine balance at times."

The Pharmaceutical Manufacturers Association remains undaunted. Insisting that the drug industry is not the problem but part of the solution to rising health care costs, industry officials say nothing else in the medical system is as cost effective as drugs.

Who believes that it's not worth spending $3 a day to escape heart surgery, or $365 for a contraceptive implant to prevent pregnancy, or $150 for vaccinations that will protect against more than a half dozen childhood diseases, they ask. Certainly not people like John Forrest, Jr., the Philadelphia electrician who remembers the precise time when a $2,200 drug shut off his heart attack.

But that isn't really the question. Everyone agrees that life, good health, and freedom from pain are worth almost anything. No question about their value.

The question is: What is a fair price and who should determine it?

2.
How the drug industry woos doctors

Dressed in a pin-striped suit and wearing highly polished black shoes, Jim Purcell was staking out the drug supply closet of a clinic at the University of Pennsylvania Medical Center. Doctors rushed by the salesman for Stuart Pharmaceuticals, going in and out of the supply room to get medicine for indigent patients. Purcell stood nearby, waiting for his chance.

His goal this day was to convince some of these doctors that a drug made by his company was the best choice for certain heart patients. So far, though, the doctors weren't stopping to hear his pitch. Now he stepped in quickly to strike up a conversation with Eric Aguiar, a senior resident. Moving deftly to stay out of the way of fast-moving doctors, Purcell listened politely as Aguiar observed that his company's hypertension drug, Zestril, seemed to be very expensive. . . .

Jim Purcell is one of the 45,000 sales representatives who hover about the doctors of this country, trying to convince physicians that theirs is the best of all possible drugs.

The sales reps are everywhere. The typical American doctor sees two or three a week. And for many doctors, the sales rep is the primary source of information on new drugs. Drug company promotion is likely to have more of an effect on what brand-name drug a doctor prescribes—

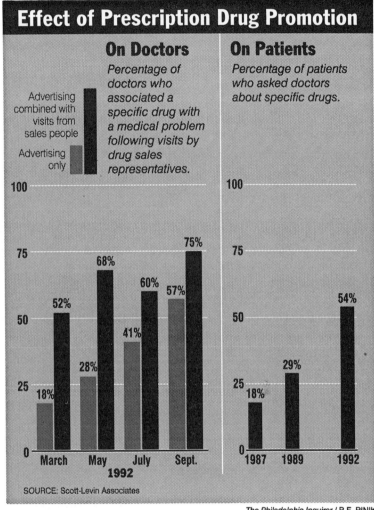

Effect of Prescription Drug Promotion

On Doctors

Percentage of doctors who associated a specific drug with a medical problem following visits by drug sales representatives.

Advertising combined with visits from sales people

Advertising only

On Patients

Percentage of patients who asked doctors about specific drugs.

On Doctors chart:
- March: 18%, 52%
- May: 28%, 68%
- July: 41%, 60%
- Sept.: 57%, 75%

1992

On Patients chart:
- 1987: 18%
- 1989: 29%
- 1992: 54%

SOURCE: Scott-Levin Associates

The Philadelphia Inquirer / B.F. BINIK

and what the patient pays—than the doctor's education or all the technical articles in medical journals.

This army of salespeople—one for every twelve prescribing doctors in the nation—is one reason prescription drug prices in the United States are so high. And it is just one of the ways in which the pharmaceutical industry exerts influence over the medical system in America.

The influence is by no means limited to doctors, although roughly 75 percent of drug companies' promotion efforts are aimed at doctors.

Drug companies also work hard to influence pharmacists, nurses, and hospital administrators, who along with doctors determine which drugs are chosen for the formulary, the official list of drugs to be prescribed within any institution.

Drug companies control practically all information on new drugs; they also influence some articles appearing in medical journals. They sponsor seminars and specialized follow-up courses for doctors. They court legislators, consumer groups, and even patients, via a barrage of drug advertising on TV. Few consumers are wooed as intensively, though, as doctors are pursued by the pharmaceutical industry.

It begins the moment a medical student starts school and receives a free stethoscope, compliments of a drug manufacturer. And it doesn't let up until the doctor retires, many thousands of prescriptions later. Sales reps routinely hand out memo pads, pens, and other "reminder" items to keep the names of their drugs before the physician. They often pay for pizza and hoagie lunches provided to hospital staffs during departmental meetings.

"Drug companies have established an amazing presence in our medical system," said Frederick Fenster, a Seattle internist and a professor at the University of Washington. "Their influence is everywhere. They are present at nearly all educational meetings for doctors and help subsidize virtually all postgraduate educational offerings."

"It's probably shocking to people who don't know, to find out the almost total control that the pharmaceutical industry has about the flow of information," said Kenneth Feather, head of surveillance and enforcement for the Food and Drug Administration's drug-marketing division.

At stake is $55 billion a year that prescription drug manufacturers make in U.S. sales. All but about $5 billion of that goes to big, brand-name companies, members of the Pharmaceutical Manufacturers Association.

About twenty cents of every dollar you spend on brand-name drugs goes to promote and market them. Companies collectively spend more than $10 billion a year on promotion in the United States—more than they spend here on research and development.

More than $3 billion a year is spent on sales representatives alone. The largest U.S. drug firm, Merck & Co., for example, spends more than $125,000 for each salesperson, according to Hemant Shah, a financial analyst who closely follows the industry. With 2,700 reps, that means Merck's U.S. sales force cost roughly $337 million in 1991.

The industry spends more than a half-billion dollars for ads in the nation's medical journals and billions more for other sales activities. Consumers finance all this promotion, through drug prices. Because most of this effort is directed at about 550,000 prescribing physicians, it means that about $13,000 a year is being spent *per doctor* to influence the medical treatment you get.

Working the general medical clinic at Penn is difficult because of restrictions imposed on sales representatives, who must sign up months in advance. They are allowed to stay in the clinic only thirty minutes—they have to make way for the next sales rep on the list—and can't stray more than a few feet from the medical supply room, which contains all the free samples that reps leave for doctors.

Standing near the door, Purcell listened politely to Eric Aguiar's comments about high prices, and thanked the doctor for his concern. Then, the pitch.

Purcell said his company's hypertension drug, Zestril, had a big advantage over some competitors': It is taken only once a day, while some competing drugs require two or more doses. The more often a patient has to take a pill, the more likely the patient is to forget. Having caught Aguiar's attention, Purcell pressed ahead. He said his company, a unit of ICI Americas, offered patients using Zestril money-saving coupons, free products, and a monthly health newsletter.

Purcell said later that he was particularly happy about working in a hospital like Penn's and for a chance to talk to resident physicians who will soon be going into private practice. "Being a teaching hospital, they go out of the university program to practices and fellowships," Purcell said. "If they use Zestril here, there is a pretty good chance they will use it out there."

When physicians write prescriptions, most patients assume their doctor chooses the drug on the basis of scientific research, wisdom, and a fine education. But it doesn't quite happen that way.

Doctors are taught only general principles of pharmacology in medical school classes. Most of their practical knowledge about drugs comes in hospital training with practicing physicians, whose choices often are influenced by which drugs are on their medical center's formulary. That, in turn, is influenced by the marketing skills of drug companies.

That's why prescribing habits vary so much between equally well-informed doctors. A doctor treating arthritis may prescribe Voltaren if he trained at Hospital A and Naprosyn if he trained at Hospital B. That's because Hospital A's formulary lists Voltaren as its primary choice for arthritis, and Hospital B stocks Naprosyn.

More than 2,500 prescription drugs are available, and new ones constantly are introduced. Most doctors are familiar with a relatively small number. The average generalist is familiar with about fifty drugs, doctors say. So they rely on drug company reps and industry-sponsored

What Doctors Don't Know About Prescription Drug Prices

132 doctors were asked to estimate the cost of specific amounts of drugs in a 1992 study by the University of Massachusetts and Harvard University.

Drug	Actual Price	Physician Estimate
Ampicillin	$7.33	$12.12
Cardizem	$52.19	$58.62
Cipro	$76.44	$54.15
Dyazide	$31.28	$27.49
Furosemide	$8.48	$16.86
Isodril	$20.74	$28.61
Isosorbide	$5.43	$20.67
Lasix	$16.98	$27.81
Micro-K	$16.08	$26.78
Naprosyn	$59.93	$41.45
Potassium chloride elixir	$4.28	$5.33
Procardia	$44.90	$54.28
Tenormin	$65.63	$47.25
Zantac	$76.18	$52.58

SOURCE: Gerontology Institute, University of Massachusetts.

The Philadelphia Inquirer / B.F. BINIK

seminars to keep up. Although formal medical education may give physicians a grounding for choosing one class of drugs for a particular problem, there's often little science behind the choice of one brand-name drug over another.

Doctors know even less about drug *costs*. A 1992 study by the University of Massachusetts and Harvard Medical School found "a widespread ignorance" about the cost of drugs by doctors and yet a high level of agreement that the affordability of a drug should be considered in prescribing.

What this means is that some checks and balances that help keep prices in line on other products are missing on prescription drugs. First, the sales pitch is made not to the purchaser but to the doctor, who makes the buying decision for the patient. The doctor's primary concern is effectiveness, not price. Second, the patient acquiesces in the choice, thinking the doctor wouldn't prescribe an expensive drug if it weren't necessary. What the patient doesn't realize is that the doctor, like anyone else, is susceptible to drug industry advertising.

Drug advertising is no different from any other advertising, except for one point, said Dr. Douglas R. Waud, who teaches pharmacology at the University of Massachusetts Medical School. "With drugs, the person who writes the order is not the person who pays the bill."

The dependence of doctors on drug companies for information is not new, but the size of the sales force is. Between 1980 and 1990, the number of sales representatives increased by 40 percent, so that today some 45,000 salespeople—"detailers," in industry jargon—roam the country buttonholing doctors, according to Scott-Levin Associates of Newtown, Bucks County, Pa., a pharmaceutical marketing service. "This reliance on detail men is disturbing, particularly since in 1988 less than 5 percent of these people had formal training in pharmacology," said the Massachusetts-Harvard report.

How much of a difference do sales reps make? Consider what happened with Augmentin, an antibiotic often prescribed for children's ear infections.

When the drug was launched on the American market by the Beecham Group in late 1984, the British firm fielded a 600-person sales force, a relatively small staff. By 1988, U.S. sales were $164 million a year—a respectable showing but not a blockbuster drug.

One year later, Beecham merged with SmithKline Beckman Corp. of Philadelphia. The U.S. sales force more than tripled, to 2,000. By the end of 1991, annual U.S. sales had almost tripled, to $400 million. "Ninety-nine-and-a-half percent" of Augmentin's success can be traced to frequent physician office visits by the sales force, said Roger W. Baker, a vice president at SmithKline.

And the price? Augmentin now sells wholesale for $51.90 for 30 tablets, more than double the price when the drug debuted in 1984.

In England, the primary drug reference book for doctors is *MIMS* (*Monthly Index of Medical Specialties*). No family practitioner's office is without it. A paperback book of 320 pages, it is slightly larger and thicker than *Reader's Digest*.

It is dwarfed by the most frequently used reference in the United States, the *Physicians' Desk Reference*, a large, hardcover book with 2,500 pages. The *Physicians' Desk Reference*, which costs $57.95 retail, is mailed free to 500,000 practicing physicians. Drug firms pay up to $12,000 a page to be listed; drugs of the few brand-name firms that choose not to pay are not listed.

MIMS in England makes it easy for doctors to compare drugs. Each entry, about the size of a program highlight on the TV page, is listed

Where Doctors Get Their Drug Information

American: Physicians' Desk Reference (PDR).

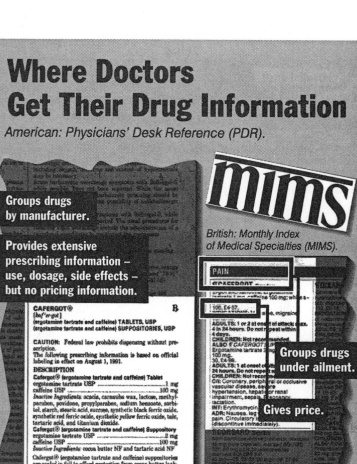

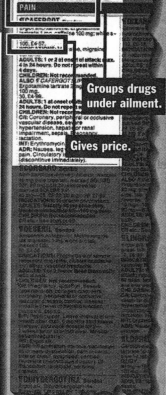

Groups drugs by manufacturer.

Provides extensive prescribing information – use, dosage, side effects – but no pricing information.

British: Monthly Index of Medical Specialties (MIMS).

PAIN

Groups drugs under ailment.

Gives price.

CAFERGOT®

(ergotamine tartrate and caffeine) TABLETS, USP
(ergotamine tartrate and caffeine) SUPPOSITORIES, USP

CAUTION: Federal law prohibits dispensing without prescription.
The following prescribing information is based on official labeling in effect on August 1, 1991.

DESCRIPTION

Cafergot® (ergotamine tartrate and caffeine) Tablet
ergotamine tartrate USP .... 1 mg
caffeine USP .... 100 mg

PDR® 46 EDITION 1992

Continued on next page

The Philadelphia Inquirer / B. F. BINIK

according to the medical problem it is designed to treat. And each entry includes the cost of the drug.

The *Physicians' Desk Reference* lists drugs by brand name and under the names of their manufacturer, a layout that is useful for doctors looking up specific drugs or manufacturers but cumbersome for those wanting to compare one product with another. The listings include all side effects and label information required by the Food and Drug Administration and can run several columns of type for each drug. But one fact is conspicuously missing: price.

A U.S. version of *MIMS* introduced in 1985 is gaining popularity among physicians. Called the *Monthly Prescribing Reference,* the book is almost identical to *MIMS* except for one thing. It contains no pricing information.

As a senior regulatory review officer for the U.S. Food and Drug Administration, David Banks bird-dogged drug companies—poring over advertisements, screening television spots, and ferreting out underhanded promotional tactics.

He helped uncover misleading information distributed by a company suggesting that an arthritis medicine might also prevent joint degeneration. He stopped another company from distributing promotional material disguised as a medical publication. "The pharmaceutical industry undertakes many, many drug promotional activities that appear to be anything but drug promotion," Banks said.

The disguises are many, he said:

- A drug company may write an article about a medicine, find a physician willing to accept authorship, and find a medical journal to publish it.
- A drug company may subsidize a doctor who lectures at medical conferences through an "educational grant." The physician is chosen because he or she is known to favor a particular drug.
- A drug company may pay physicians to test a new medicine on patients. It is called a post-marketing drug study but serves as an incentive for the doctor to prescribe the medicine.

As for the reliability of print advertising, 60 percent of drug ads in medical journals reviewed were rated "poor or unacceptable" in a 1992 study prepared for the inspector general's office of the U.S. Department of Health and Human Services.

Banks said the entangled relationship between the industry and medical community leads to misleading information. "Drug company financial relationships with the research and physician communities have become so widespread, and drug company control over public discussions of drug therapy so pervasive, that literally any public discussion of drugs should be considered potentially subject to drug company bias."

Banks, who said he was disappointed with the impact of his efforts, has decided to leave after more than four years of trying to regulate drug industry advertising.

There is strong evidence to suggest that drug promotional activities:

- Create a physician loyalty so that the brand-name drug will retain a chunk of the market years after patents have expired and cheaper generics have arrived. Example: Valium is still one of the most popular tranquilizers, even though it costs up to seven times more than chemically identical generic products.
- Encourage physicians to prescribe drugs, when cheaper and safer treatments are available. Example: Doctors often prescribe cholesterol-lowering drugs, even though they know most patients can—and should—reduce cholesterol levels through diet and exercise. Both the industry and physicians say they tell patients to try diet and exercise first. Then they prescribe pills. The cholesterol drug Mevacor, on the market since 1987, has become the ninth-best-selling drug in the world.

Although doctors insist commercial interests do not affect their medical judgment, Jerry Avorn of the Harvard Medical School in a 1982 study concluded that promotional activities were far more important in determining what drugs were prescribed than doctors realized or cared to admit.

Avorn surveyed 85 primary-care physicians in the Boston area, and most, as expected, said sales reps and pharmaceutical advertisements were "minimally" important in influencing their prescribing habits. Then Avorn asked whether they agreed with either of these statements: that propoxyphene (Darvon) was a more effective pain reliever than aspirin, and that mental failure in the elderly was the result of inadequate blood flow to the brain because of hardening of cerebral arteries.

One-third of those surveyed believed that drugs relieved confusion in elderly patients by dilating cerebral arteries, and 49 percent thought Darvon was a better pain reliever than aspirin. The questions were tricks, designed to find out how much the doctors were being influenced by pharmaceutical advertising. Only drug ads had suggested that Darvon was a superior pain reliever and that narrowed cerebral arteries lead to mental failure in the elderly. The scientific literature did not show this.

"Although the vast majority of practitioners perceived themselves as paying little attention to drug advertisments and detail men," Avorn concluded, the study "revealed quite the opposite pattern of influence in large segments of the sample."

Why are doctors so readily influenced?

"Drug advertisements," Avorn wrote, "are simply more visually arresting and conceptually accessible than are papers in the medical literature, and physicians appear to respond to the difference." In other words, advertising works with physicians just as it does with everyone else.

Dr. Douglas Waud says there's no free lunch—and doctors ought to know it. In a July 30, 1992, article in the *New England Journal of Medicine,* the University of Massachusetts Medical School professor had this to say about drug industry promotion:

"From the press, one can get an idea of what it costs to buy a judge or a senator—generally, thousands of dollars. But you can buy a physician for a pen or some pizza and beer for a departmental meeting. . . . Am I supposed to believe that the members of a clinical department are so impoverished that they cannot buy their own pens or pizza and beer?

"It is amazing how dull-witted some of my colleagues can be in this regard. One division chief went around for weeks with a shirt-pocket protector holding his collection of pens and displaying an advertisement for a drug. These plastic pouches cost about fifty cents. The 'gift' was of trivial value. Yet the man was willing to be a walking billboard for this meager reward. . . .

"So where does this [promotion] money come from? Obviously, it comes out of the pockets of patients. . . . It does not come from the tooth fairy. Accepting these bribes therefore boils down to cheating patients. . . .

"I can see that it is appropriate for the telephone company to try to persuade us to use the telephone more. I cannot see that it is appropriate for a drug company to get us to prescribe a drug we would not otherwise prescribe. The party line, of course, is that the advertising provides education. If you were buying a used car, would you get your information from Sam, the friendly used-car salesman?"

The influence of drug companies on the medical system became so pervasive that Congress became concerned. In 1990, Congress held hearings on the promotional activities of the industry. And in 1991, the Food and Drug Administration moved to put limits on some industry activities.

Most of the attention focused on continuing medical education and other programs designed to keep doctors up to date. The government and some professional organizations, such as the American Medical Association and the American College of Physicians, were concerned about industry-sponsored educational seminars and dinners. These were often held in elegant hotels or resort centers, with speakers and programs selected by the drug company sponsoring the event. The industry also was underwriting many accredited courses for doctors, one- or two-day seminars held at academic centers and taught by specialists.

"This practice of underwriting offerings of academic organizations and institutions creates the opportunity for the often subtle introduction of commercially oriented content," a statement by the American College of Physicians published in 1990 said.

Just how incestuous the relationship had become was described by David C. Jones, a former public relations executive for Ciba-Geigy and Abbott Laboratories, at 1990 hearings before the U.S. Senate Committee on Labor and Human Resources, headed by Sen. Edward M. Kennedy (D., Mass.).

"Medical education is now determined by what the marketing department wants, not what doctors need. Doctors themselves are recruited to publish helpful articles which are produced by company medical writers, who assure that the marketing messages are featured prominently."

Jones also said: "Consumer demand is created routinely through the news media. Print and broadcast outlets are flooded with packaged stories and TV productions that target doctors and consumers. Prescription drugs are marketed as if they were cosmetics or candy. Claims are made beyond what the product will do. Demand is inflated beyond the medical need. Uses are promoted that are neither healthy nor wise."

The Food and Drug Administration, under the direction of David Kessler, sought to clearly detail in a policy statement activities that required regulatory oversight. The agency wanted to make sure companies could not disguise promotional efforts in supposedly independent programs, such as continuing medical education courses. The agency released a draft of a nineteen-page concept paper in the autumn of 1991 that outlined how that would be done. The fallout was immediate.

James Todd, executive vice president of the American Medical Association, agreed that "there has been a blurring of the line between education and promotion in many programs." But the AMA and other physician groups said the proposed federal policy constituted "micromanagement" and intruded on the profession's own regulatory structure.

While the federal agency was still considering its policy statement, the AMA's ethics committee worked up more specific guidance on doctors' acceptance of gifts from industry. The doctors would police themselves.

The drug industry became less free with its money, waiting to see what would unfold.

The Food and Drug Administration's proposed policy "would have killed" continuing medical education, Gerald J. Mossinghoff, executive director of the Pharmaceutical Manufacturers Association, said in an interview in September 1992.

"It got the government totally involved. We are the accused, and they are the cops with CME [continuing medical education]. That was opposed, not only by us but a lot of sensible people on the Hill. And a lot of others. That was why it was so drastically changed and, in effect, withdrawn. Those were bad ideas."

The AMA's more specific instructions about acceptance of gifts didn't go down too well, either. "Several specialty societies criticized the AMA document as too specific and insulting physicians' ability to know right from wrong," AMA general counsel Kirk Johnson said in 1992. The AMA ethics committee revised the instructions.

The Food and Drug Administration, under heavy pressure, reworked the concept paper. "They substantially revised it," Johnson said. "We believe it was held up by the [Bush] administration. It was concerned whether the FDA was adding to the regulatory burden to the general physician and drug companies."

The federal agency released a draft of a new policy statement on November 27, 1992. The policy leaves the monitoring of continuing medical education to private accrediting organizations, with the Food and Drug Administration stepping in only if necessary.

"As the FDA began to see what the private sector was doing, they saw that their concerns were being addressed," Todd of the American Medical Association said. "We are happy with the changes they have made. . . . We believe the FDA would like to see this handled in the private sector and not get involved in detailed enforcement."

Some doctors say the educational seminars now appear to be more independent. Nicole Lurie, a Minneapolis physician who had testified at the Senate hearings, recently said she sees fewer "strings attached."

The AMA seems now to realize that the gift of education is not purely altruistic. When asked whether it wouldn't be cleaner if drug firms simply contributed to an educational pool, as some have suggested, so that their influence couldn't be attached to a given course, AMA trustee Nancy Dickey said: "I have heard discussions of blind funding of courses, but one of the downsides is: Why would the pharmaceutical companies contribute to blind funding at all?"

"We are not philanthropic organizations," said J.P. Garnier, president of North American pharmaceutical operations for SmithKline Beecham. "We derive goodwill from funding continuing medical education programs with our customer base. If we had to pool with other companies, then the goodwill would be lost."

The medical system has become so dependent on the pharmaceutical marketing system that many programs for doctors would be threatened if the industry cut back its promotion dollars—and the industry knows it. If drug industry money weren't available, "there would be a lot less education out there," said Andy Anderson, president of U.S. pharmaceuticals for G.D. Searle & Co.

And hospital staffs would have to start buying their own pastrami sandwiches.

Arthur M. Zoloth, director of pharmacy at Virginia Mason Medical Center in Seattle, was telling the Senate committee hearings about the many ways the drug industry had tried to befriend him.

It started in pharmacy school, when the industry gave him complimentary subscriptions to newsletters, travel expenses to visit drug companies, and sent a graduation gift. Early in his career, he lunched with drug company sales staff. Few lunches provided important information on medicines, he said.

"It wasn't until I was the recipient of a gold-plated paperweight depicting a chicken egg, as an inducement to buy flu vaccine, that I came to the realization that these marketing tactics were expensive and ultimately the cost would be borne by the patient," he said. "I felt a sense of frustration and anger with an industry that wastes resources while appearing to be insensitive to the cost of drugs to patients. Subsequently, I stopped accepting the marketing trinkets."

Trinkets aside, Zoloth has served as a consultant on advisory boards for several drug firms and two manufacturers of intravenous solutions. "While I would like to believe these appointments were based solely on my intellect," he said, "I cannot help but feel they may have been based upon my perceived purchasing authority."

Formularies are the master lists of approved drugs for medical institutions. The pharmacists, doctors, nurses, and administrators who serve on the committees that select which drugs will go on the formulary are very important to drug companies.

Scott-Levin Associates, the Newtown, Pa., pharmaceutical marketing service, surveyed seventy-four HMO pharmacy directors during an eight-week period in the spring of 1992 and found that drug company representatives had made more than 2,200 visits. That's thirty visits per director, almost four a week. "They are trying to establish a relationship, as they do with a physician," said Jeff Long, a Scott-Levin official.

One reason that getting on the formularies is all-important: They serve as marketing tools.

J.P. Garnier, president of SmithKline Beecham pharmaceutical operations in North America, acknowledged in a 1991 public hearing in Harrisburg, Pa., that his company gives deep discounts to Kaiser Permanente, one of the nation's largest health maintenance organizations.

"The hope is that even though our [discounted] product will not be very profitable in the hands of Kaiser Permanente, when those same physicians move to other institutions, they will have experience with our drugs and use them more extensively than the competition," Garnier said in an interview. "Therefore, to some extent, the discounts to Kaiser serve as an investment for the future."

Discounts are something the industry does not talk much about. But as purchasing groups have grown, they have used their buying clout to force price deals for their members. The growth of these managed-care groups, and drug companies' need to get their medicines on the formularies, are spurring a kind of price competition that drug-makers previously haven't had to face. Until recently, it was the companies that could pick and choose to whom they would grant discounts.

The companies have been particularly generous with drugs sold to the Veterans Administration (now the Department of Veterans Affairs), and for good reason. More than 50 percent of all physicians in the United States have had training at the VA's 170 hospitals, according to the agency.

"There's a tremendous commercial advantage for companies to introduce their products to the physician at a time when they are forming their therapeutic habits," Garnier said at the hearing in Harrisburg. For instance, he said, SmithKline knows that if veterans hospitals carry its flagship ulcer medicine, Tagamet, 50 percent of the doctors will learn about it.

Companies will fight for the opportunity. Look at what happened at the Hospital of the University of Pennsylvania in the spring of 1990:

A hospital formulary committee decided that patients who needed an ulcer drug would get Tagamet because SmithKline offered the best deal through the hospital's buying group. The pharmacy saved about $200,000 a year, a 33 percent reduction from the previous year, said Jeffrey Bourret, the hospital's director of pharmacy. He said the hospital felt comfortable using Tagamet because the committee had determined it is essentially the same as three rival products: Zantac made by Glaxo of London, Pepcid made by Merck & Co. of Rahway, N.J., and Axid made by Eli Lilly & Co. of Indianapolis.

The edict was simple: Once the drug went onto the formulary, doctors had to prescribe Tagamet when their patients needed an ulcer medicine. If, for some reason, the SmithKline drug didn't agree with a patient, the physician had another choice: Merck's Pepcid. The Glaxo and Lilly drugs were out of contention.

The Glaxo people were not happy. Zantac once had most of the hospital's ulcer business.

"There was an attempt to undermine the decision of the pharmacy and therapeutics committee," Bourret said. According to him, Glaxo sales reps persuaded a number of hospital doctors to write letters, objecting to the committee's decision. Their contention was that Zantac was a better drug.

Bourret said the hospital committee had been "painstaking" in reaching a decision, drawing on advice of expert physicians and other medical staff. Even so, he said, the hospital had to wipe out the misinformation spread by Glaxo before it could implement the formulary. The hospital sent the drug company a letter of reprimand.

Rick Sluder, a spokesman for Glaxo, said: "It is true that our representative in the hospital spoke with physicians who were dissatisfied with the committee's decision. And she supported their efforts to make their dissatisfaction known to the committee. They felt inclusion on the formulary was important to patient care. . . . We received a letter that further suggested the hospital shouldn't be divided over the issue. Glaxo should do nothing to contribute to devisiveness. In our view, we weren't."

A footnote: In 1992, Glaxo's Zantac was put on the formulary as the second choice behind SmithKline's Tagamet. Bourret said the drug was cheaper than Merck's Pepcid.

Abbey Meyers considers herself a homemaker, not a lobbyist. But in certain circles, she is well known for her long fight to make sure affordable medicine is available for patients who have long been ignored.

Meyers, executive director of the National Organization for Rare Disorders, was drawn out of her cozy suburban home in the early 1980s, not long after her oldest child was diagnosed with a neurological disorder called Tourette syndrome. Her son was receiving a new drug on an experimental basis, she said. When it became clear that the drug would not make it to market for the treatment of schizophrenia—a more prevalent disease, with a larger potential market—the company lost interest, Meyers said.

"Anger is not the word. I was irate," she said. "In society, we talk about compassion. . . . How could we allow this to happen to a living child? It didn't make sense."

Meyers, who was then a board member of the Tourette Syndrome Association, wrote letters to everybody—drug companies, politicians, the Food and Drug Administration, consumer groups.

The companies generally didn't develop or market drugs for rare diseases like her son's. It simply wasn't profitable. So Abbey Meyers helped push for legislation that would give a financial incentive to companies to develop drugs for small patient groups. President Reagan signed the Orphan Drug Act in 1983.

The law gives a company exclusive rights to market its drug for seven years without competition and provides tax credits. But some companies profiteered under the protection of the law. In late 1991 and early '92, Meyers and others lobbied Congress to amend the law to allow competition once total sales from an orphan drug reached $200 million. Suddenly, Abbey Meyers found herself and her organization under attack.

"A friend who is well placed within the drug industry said to us, 'Watch yourself. I hear rumors that you will be the object of dirty tricks,'" said Dr. Jess Thoene, president of the group, which represents 127 voluntary health groups. "I took the warning seriously."

So did some of Meyers's professional colleagues. "Some voluntary health agencies, including some of our members, were afraid if they vocally supported the revisions in the Orphan Drug Act, they would lose donations from pharmaceutical companies," Meyers said. "So they sat on the fence and became neutral."

The revisions have not been passed.

Nothing happens on Capitol Hill affecting the drug industry without the input—some say resistance—of the Pharmaceutical Manufacturers Association.

Working out of elegant offices several blocks from the White House, the trade group spends $31 million a year pushing the industry's case. It is considered one of the most powerful lobbying organizations in Washington, along with the American Medical Association and the National Rifle Association, and can take much of the credit for killing or watering down legislation the industry doesn't like.

No legislative hearing involving drugs is so insignificant as not to have a pharmaceutical industry representative in attendance, amply supplied with industry-generated statistics and literature that deliver essentially the same message: Prescription drugs are cost-effective, account for only 7 percent of the medical care costs in this country, and

How Top 10 Recipients of Drug PAC Money Voted

Senator David Pryor (D., Ark.) sponsored a bill that would link a lucrative federal tax break for U.S. companies operating in Puerto Rico with stable prices. This vote was to table the bill – and thus kill it.

VOTE TO TABLE	1981-91 DRUG INDUSTRY CONTRIBUTIONS	
YES	NO	
✓		Orrin G. Hatch (R., Utah) — $120,162
✓		Bill Bradley (D., N.J.) — $99,707
✓		Daniel R. Coats (R., Ind.) — $99,300
✓		Dave Durenberger (R., Minn.) — $96,702
✓		Phil Gramm (R., Tex.) — $80,332
	✓	Arlen Specter (R., Pa.) — $73,650
✓		Frank R. Lautenberg (D., N.J.) — $72,150
✓		John H. Chafee (R., R.I.) — $56,650
✓		Charles E. Grassley (R., Iowa) — $56,650
✓		Steve Symms (R., Idaho) — $56,033

The Philadelphia Inquirer / B.F. BINIK

shouldn't come under too much regulation. It costs $231 million to bring a drug to market, and the industry has to make a sizable profit to reward its investors for taking risks.

To sustain its position, the industry spreads campaign money through its political action committees to key senators and members of Congress—$8 million between 1981 and 1991, according to a study by the public advocacy group Common Cause. That was a healthy part of the $60 million contributed by all of the medical-industry political action committees.

The Pharmaceutical Manufacturers Association's lobbying has proved highly effective.

In 1991, Sen. David Pryor of Arkansas introduced a bill that tied lucrative tax breaks for U.S. pharmaceutical companies operating in Puerto Rico to price inflation. If prices of a company's products exceeded the rate of inflation, the company's tax benefit would be reduced. The bill was one the drug industry obviously did not want. For eight hours in March 1992, the Senate debated the proposal. Then, for the first time ever, the full U.S. Senate voted on a bill to impose price controls on pharmaceuticals in the private market. The vote was 61–36—to table the bill.

Here's how the top ten recipients of drug-company money voted and what they said during floor debate:

"Prescription drugs represent 7 percent of our total health-care expenditures," said John H. Chafee (R., R.I.), who voted to table. "Let us wrestle with the other parts . . . that make up that 93 percent of health care costs which is not represented by drugs." The drug industry contributed $56,650 to Chafee's campaigns between 1981 and 1991.

"It costs $231 million to develop a main-line drug today, and we are developing them right and left in this country because of the incentives," said Orrin G. Hatch (R., Utah), who voted to table. The drug industry contributed $120,162 to his campaigns between 1981 and 1991.

"It could have significant and adverse effects on the future discovery of breakthrough drugs, and the growth of an industry that has been one of the bright spots on our economic horizon," said Frank R. Lautenberg (D., N.J.), who voted to table. The drug industry contributed $72,150 to his campaigns between 1981 and 1991.

"Certainly, lower prices will help consumers to be able to afford prescription drugs," said Bill Bradley (D., N.J.). "But the question is, what are they going to be able to buy? If you asked those whose lives have been saved due to innovations in the pharmaceutical industry, price controls may not be pro-consumer." He voted to table. The drug industry contributed $99,707 to his campaigns between 1981 and 1991.

"In a nutshell, the result of this amendment would be to increase drug prices, harm the economy of Puerto Rico, negatively affect tax incentives, and weaken the United States patent system," said Steve Symms (R., Idaho), who opposed the bill. The drug industry contributed $56,033 to his campaigns between 1981 and 1991.

"If socialism worked, we would have torn down the Berlin Wall to reach to the other side," said Phil Gramm (R., Tex.). "It did not work, so they tore it down to get to our side. Why do we want to impose price controls?" He voted to table. The drug industry contributed $80,332 to his campaigns between 1981 and 1991.

"My opposition to this amendment should in no way be construed as condoning the pricing practices of the pharmaceutical industry," said David Durenberger (R., Minn.). "I am pledged to find market-based solutions to the problems of escalating drug prices." He voted to table. The drug industry contributed $96,702 to his campaigns between 1981 and 1991.

"It is important to understand that in preserving this industry we are affecting our economy in a number of ways, but more importantly, we are bringing some very real advances in the diagnosis and treatment—particularly in the treatment—of disease and illness to the American people and in fact to the people of the world," said Daniel R. Coats (R., Ind.). He voted to table. The drug industry contributed $99,300 to his campaigns between 1981 and 1991.

Charles E. Grassley (R., Iowa) did not speak during the debate. He voted to table. The drug industry contributed $58,250 to his campaigns between 1981 and 1991.

Arlen Specter (R., Pa.), who received $73,650, voted against tabling. He did not speak during the debate. Although he had some problems with the bill, he supported Pryor's efforts to control prescription drug price inflation, Specter's spokeswoman, Susan Lamontagne, said.

"We had seventeen senators—from both parties—who spoke up forcefully and made the right points for the right reasons," said Paul Freiman, chief executive officer of Syntex Corp. and chairman of the Pharmaceutical Manufacturers Association. "They recognized our contributions to the U.S. economy, the value of our R&D spending, and our role as the most cost-effective segment of health care expenditures."

The drug industry gets direct access to members of Congress, said Meyers of the National Organization for Rare Disorders, an advocate for lower drug prices. "We don't. If you have given a substantial contribution . . . the door is always open. They can go with their fancy accounting figures [on how drugs supposedly save patients money], and the senator doesn't question it. Because the congressmen take their word for it, they all get up and repeat the same line."

This wasn't the only victory for the pharmaceutical lobbyists in 1992. Among the legislation they successfully opposed was a bill that would eliminate monopoly protection provided under the Orphan Drug Act once a drug's sales had passed $200 million. Several senators prevented the bill from coming to a vote by the full Senate. Another bill, the Health Care Cost Containment and Reform Act, included provisions to establish an outpatient prescription drug benefit under Medicare with limits for the amount the government would pay for pills. The bill was not voted on in the 102d Congress.

Congress did vote on one bill opposed by most of the industry. It requires the drug industry to grant discounts for prescription drug purchases by government veterans hospitals, Department of Defense medical facilities, and some public health clinics. The bill was passed, but drug industry lobbyists succeeded in preventing inclusion of a price-control provision the industry strongly opposed. It was signed into law in November 1992.

Many medical groups tread gingerly when it comes to challenging the drug industry about high drug costs. Each organization has its own special concerns.

Cancer drugs are among the costliest in the nation. A spokesman for the American Society of Clinical Oncologists, which represents cancer specialists, said dwindling federal funding has increased the importance of the research money its members get from the pharmaceutical industry.

"Sure, we'd like to see prices go down as much as possible," said the group's lobbyist, Stacey Beckhardt, "but not at the expense of a legitimate source of funding for research."

The American Heart Association was instrumental in getting the industry to launch a program of free drugs to patients who can't afford them. The program was started after the association published a report in October 1991 about people who couldn't afford expensive cardiovascular drugs.

"If you try to investigate the high price of drugs in this country and tried to do something about it, that would postpone getting medicine to the people who needed it because the pharmaceutical industry would not be cooperative," said Harriet P. Dustan, chairwoman of the committee that did the report on heart patients.

One of the few major professional groups that has been willing to talk with the drug industry about lowering prices is the American Medical Association. In a masterfully balanced resolution in 1991, the AMA House of Delegates voted to ask the Pharmaceutical Manufacturers Association to "enter into a dialogue" on ways to reduce prices "through such mechanisms as cost-effective research and development" and "more modest promotional activities"—two suggestions the drug industry group would undoubtedly debate—and "product liability reform" and "streamlining FDA requirements for new drug approvals"—two suggestions the organization would eagerly endorse. But the dialogue has been limited, said the AMA's Kirk Johnson.

Reform may be in the wind. In September 1992, the American College of Physicians, the nation's second-largest physician group, called for a major overhaul of the U.S. health care system, including placing a cap on national health spending and putting "realistic" limits on doctors' fees. The plan does not single out drug costs but seeks to reform the entire medical system.

"The profession is just beginning to get serious about overall costs," said H. Denman Scott, senior vice president of health and public policy in the College of Physicians.

Why has it taken so long for the medical profession to confront this problem?

"I don't think there's been enough pressure for change," Scott said. "Not enough components of society have been saying, 'Ouch, this hurts. Help.'"

3.
Clearing the hurdles to high prices and profits

In the autumn of 1990, Congress momentarily shocked drug manufacturers by passing a law that forced them to give state Medicaid programs a discount. Since the government is the single largest purchaser of pharmaceuticals and had been paying top dollar, Congress figured it could save a lot if Medicaid got the same discount the companies were giving their best customers.

The 1990 law said the government health program for poor people must get the same price break these best customers were getting. The drug companies met this new threat in a characteristic way. They raised prices. In this case, to their best customers, effectively raising the prices they could charge Medicaid.

Turning obstacles into opportunities, and opportunities into profits—at this, the drug companies excel. No matter what hurdles are thrown in their way, they quickly adjust and recoup. And Americans end up paying more for drugs.

When Congress passed legislation intended to contain drug prices by allowing easier approval of generics, the big companies responded by raising brand-name drug prices. When big hospitals and health maintenance organizations use their clout to force price concessions, the drug companies compensate with higher prices at retail drugstores.

What Goes Into the Price of a Drug

Manufacturers' average cost breakdown.

Drug companies do not provide cost breakdowns for their drugs. This breakdown is based on studies done for the government, updated by economist Stephen Schondelmeyer.

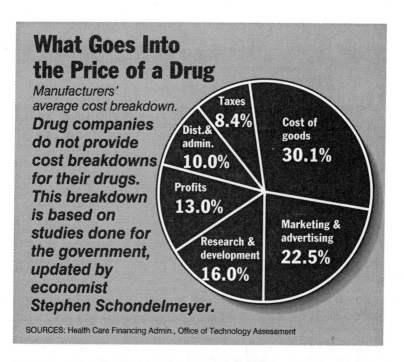

Taxes
8.4%

Dist.& admin.
10.0%

Profits
13.0%

Research & development
16.0%

Cost of goods
30.1%

Marketing & advertising
22.5%

SOURCES: Health Care Financing Admin., Office of Technology Assessment

Where Your Money Goes

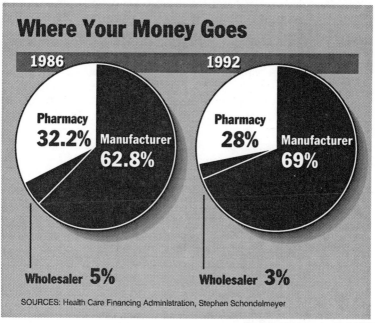

1986

Pharmacy
32.2%

Manufacturer
62.8%

Wholesaler **5%**

1992

Pharmacy
28%

Manufacturer
69%

Wholesaler **3%**

SOURCES: Health Care Financing Administration, Stephen Schondelmeyer

The Philadelphia Inquirer / B.F. BINIK

When generic drugs claimed a larger percentage of the market, brand-name companies began marketing their own generics. When manufacturers got a tax break for creating jobs in Puerto Rico, drug companies figured out how to get the best break of all.

When drug patents are about to expire, the companies make improvements in their drugs to get extra years of protection.

Whatever strategy it takes to maintain an advantage, one rule is followed: Don't reduce prices; only raise them.

"What we tend to see almost uniformly with pharmaceuticals is that their price is set and then it continues to go up," said Stephen Schondelmeyer, a University of Minnesota economist who follows the industry. "Rarely, rarely do we see prices going down."

Senator Larry Pressler (D., S.D.) calls it a system in which those with power get price breaks and those without power get soaked. "On one side, the closed market groups are given huge savings. On the other side, the pharmaceutical manufacturer charges significantly higher prices to independent pharmacies to offset the low prices in the closed market. It is a system of taking from one side in order to give to the other. Who, then, is ultimately taken? The public, of course."

Take the Medicaid case. The drug companies increased their best prices "to offset any lost revenue caused by the Medicaid drug rebate provision," the Inspector General's Office of the Department of Health and Human Services concluded in 1991. And they didn't lose any time doing it.

The Medicaid law was just a few months old when Department of Veterans Affairs officials saw some of their traditional discounts erode. Reviewing a sample of drug prices at seven VA centers after the law went into effect in 1991, a General Accounting Office report projected that "five of the seven centers will experience cost increases from 8 to 11 percent. The other centers' costs will rise by 17 and 26 percent, respectively."

"While VA had anticipated some cost shifting to result from this legislation, we were surprised by its magnitude," Edward J. Derwinski, then Veterans Affairs secretary, wrote to a congressional committee.

Hospitals outside the VA system and HMOs also saw price increases. The National Association of Public Hospitals estimates that the Medicaid law cost its members more than $130 million. The largest trade association for HMOs said contract prices for individual drugs increased from 20 percent to 1,000 percent between October 1990 and April 1991.

The inspector general's report revealed that of 101 drugs reviewed, manufacturers had raised 90 of their best prices. Specifically, the review showed that thirty-seven drugs increased between 1.5 percent and 10 percent; twenty-five increased between 10 percent and 20 percent; twenty-four increased between 20 percent and 100 percent; and four drugs had increases of more than 100 percent.

"The increase in drug prices offered to hospitals, HMOs, and buying groups by the drug manufacturers has not gone unnoticed," the report concluded. "The Congress is concerned with the drug manufacturers' actions of increasing prices and their effort to shift the cost of the Medicaid rebate program to other segments of the health care industry."

For some time, high drug prices had been a problem for the fourteen health centers in the Multnomah County Health Department in Portland, Ore. Matters got worse in 1991, after Congress forced the drug companies to give price discounts to Medicaid. In one year, the price the county paid for Albuterol inhaler for asthma jumped by 157 percent. Tegretol, an epilepsy medicine, shot up 336 percent. And Norflex, a muscle relaxant, increased almost 500 percent.

"How can we provide the same level of service with these kinds of drug price increases?" asked Joy Belcourt, the health department's director of pharmacy services. "We can't increase our budget for medications based on the drug companies' needs for profits. We are somewhat captive to their medicines. We don't have a choice."

Drug company pricing strategy can be hard on individual patients, particularly older Americans with chronic conditions and no insurance.

A patient often is put on a drug in the hospital, where discounted prices have been negotiated. Once home, the patient buys the drugs at a local drugstore, which often has to pay more for drugs than anyone else in the medical care system. The reason for this is something called multitier pricing. It's a little like a water bed: Push down on prices here and they pop up over there.

Drug companies offer discounts to large buying groups, like hospitals and HMOs, which can force competitive prices. They sell drugs at reduced prices to medical centers and teaching hospitals, hoping to hook doctors into prescribing habits that carry over into their private practices. These institutions are able to force price concessions because only a limited number of drugs are on their formularies, the rosters of drugs their doctors are expected to use.

This means that patients treated in these hospitals often end up with a particular brand-name drug, not necessarily because it's better than other drugs in its class but because the hospital negotiated a good price. But all these price concessions mean that someone *else* pays—the patient, at the local drugstore. Drugstores don't get large discounts as hospitals do. The retail druggist, the primary source of drugs for most Americans, pays the highest rung on the pricing ladder.

"It is generally safe to say that the retail pharmacist is paying top dollar," said Joseph Thomas 3d, director of the pharmaceutical economics research center at Purdue University. "Generally, the independent retail pharmacist is in the weakest position" of all.

Bob Gude, president of the Pharmacy Freedom Fund, an organization of independent retail druggists, describes this process as "hooking" the patient on high-priced drugs.

"The company knows if patients are stabilized on a particular product while in the hospital that they are going to stay on the product when they get out of the hospital. So to entice the hospitals into using the product, they give them a huge discount. While it may be profitable to the hospital to use that particular brand of [medicine], over the lifetime of the patient, it is going to cost him thousands of dollars," Gude said.

The pharmaceutical industry maintains that these pricing differences reflect differences in cost, not price discrimination. "It is simply cheaper for manufacturers to do business with some organizations than with others. Discounts often reflect that fact," the Pharmaceutical Manufacturers Association wrote in 1990.

However, Will Williams, vice president of the National Wholesale Druggists' Association, pointed out that the manufacturers no longer perform most of the distribution; wholesalers do. And there is not that much difference in cost between delivering to a hospital or to a drugstore, he said.

The price difference is not always based on volume, Schondelmeyer, the University of Minnesota economist, said, because large retail drug outlets often buy more than hospitals.

The price difference, Williams said, is because drug-makers "can justify different discounts based on who can influence the use of the product." A hospital can do that better than a retail druggist.

Drug companies work with "those organizations that can put together mutually beneficial relationships. We are no different from any other industry," said Joseph Scodari, vice president and general manager of U.S. pharmaceuticals at Rhone-Poulenc Rorer.

Price concessions exist when customers are in a position to guarantee more volume or market share, he said. "If a group of pharmacists says 'We can influence what is used,' we want to negotiate. I don't think any [drug] company will walk away from a dialogue."

The Pharmacy Freedom Fund tried to organize 12,000 independent retail druggists into a buying group, but the brand-name companies wouldn't deal with them, said Joe Nellis, a lawyer formerly with the group. A similar situation occurred in Kansas when the state Medicaid program put out bids on drugs, hoping to get a pricing deal. Most brand-name drug firms declined to bid.

"The major obstacle in starting the program was the strong resistance from the major pharmaceutical companies," Winston Barton, head of the Kansas Department of Social and Rehabilitation Services, told a congressional hearing on drug prices in 1989.

It was testimony such as Barton's that led Congress to pass the Medicaid rebate in 1990. Anger over the drug industry's response to the Medicaid rebate helped push Congress into followup legislation. In the fall of 1992, Congress extended the discount requirement to several other government agencies and public health clinics.

The buyer of prescription drugs has few ways to comparison shop, unlike the case with most consumer products.

Drug firms often require big customers to sign confidential agreements not to divulge the price, said John Coster, a staff member of the Senate Special Committee on Aging. It's not just the legal threat that keeps customers quiet, according to Schondelmeyer, but also concern they could lose their favored prices. Secrecy makes it that much harder for large and small buyers to ferret out the best deal.

"If more people knew how inexpensively these medications could be made and how cheaply they are sold to other segments of the market or other parts of the world, they would be up in arms," said Tom Snedden, director of Pennsylvania's prescription drug program for low-income older people.

Manufacturers' agreements deter their customers from talking about their prices, Schondelmeyer said.

"The industry will go to all extremes to protect this uncompetitive side of the market," Coster said at a health care conference in February 1992 organized by the Wharton School of the University of Pennsylvania. "They do not want any semblance of competition from breaking down the insulated market structures [they have] created in the retail marketplace. This is the side of the market in which competition must be stimulated if we are to have any hope of controlling the cost of pharmaceuticals. But history shows that it will be difficult to do without some form of government intervention."

In the autumn of 1984, President Reagan signed legislation shortening the time it takes for cheaper generic versions of brand-name drugs to reach the market.

During a bill-signing ceremony in the Rose Garden, Reagan told guests: "Everyone wins, particularly our elderly Americans. . . . Senior citizens require more medication than any segment of our society."

The brand-name companies had opposed this legislation—sponsored by Rep. Henry A. Waxman (D., Calif.) and Sen. Orrin G. Hatch (R., Utah)—because competition from cheaper generic drugs would cost them business.

True to its promise, the Drug Price Competition and Patent Term Restoration Act brought thousands of discount medicines to market. And brand-name companies did lose customers. Studies showed that within three years after a generic came on the market, companies lost up to 50 percent of their customers.

But the other 50 percent of the patients and their doctors remained loyal to the brand names. So what did the drug companies do? They raised prices on the brand-name drugs to make up for customers they had lost. And they kept increasing prices, an average of 10.8 percent a year—four times faster than prices of generic versions, according to a study by the federal Health Care Financing Administration, which followed price increases over a seven-year period in the 1980s.

The brand-name drug often ends up being "three or five or ten, or even in some cases, twenty times the average price of the generics on the market," said Schondelmeyer, coauthor of the HCFA report.

In one extreme example, cited in the financing administration report, the price of a brand-name version of prednisone increased by 159.6 percent over the seven-year period, 72 times more than the 2.2 percent increase for generic versions. Prednisone is used to treat allergic and inflammatory conditions.

"If you look at it from a business perspective, every different approach to manage the negative impact of competition [has been tried]," said Scodari of Rhone-Poulenc Rorer. "Reducing price has been tried. Increasing price has been tried. Doing nothing has been tried. At the end of the day, the best decision is either leave price where it is or raise price. . . . The overall dollar volume is least impacted. When you drop the price to meet the generics, we can never compete with generics on price."

Many people were disappointed by the way the industry got around the Waxman-Hatch act. Among them was Hatch, a longtime ally of the industry. "I am today unconvinced that post-patent price increases, in the face of generic competition, can be justified," Hatch was quoted in a Pharmaceutical Manufacturers Association newsletter in December 1991. "In fact, such price increases appear not only to violate the fundamental principles of a free market economy, they potentially represent the most callous and insensitive abuse of customers."

Ⅰn the mountains of Puerto Rico, in a factory surrounded by palm trees and tropical plants, SmithKline Beecham makes its high-blood-pressure medicine, Dyazide. Several windowless rooms have been set aside to make batches of 11 million capsules, which are shipped to the company's mainland warehouse in Tennessee.

The medicine starts its journey when four ingredients are poured into a twelve-foot-high metal blender with a heart-shaped bowl. More than twenty drums, each weighing about 220 pounds, must be unloaded before the machine starts to rotate. Somewhat similar to sifting flour, the procedure takes thirty minutes and results in a yellow powder called Dyazide. The drug is taken down two halls into rooms where machines are filling 1,500 capsules a minute.

Some of the capsules are red and maroon, and some are white. The red and maroon capsules are sold by SmithKline Beecham under the brand name Dyazide. The white capsules are shipped to SmithKline's rival, the generic firm Rugby, which sells them under the generic designations of triamterene and hydrochlorothiazide.

Made with the exact same equipment, the exact same workers, the exact same quality control, even the exact same packaging machine, they are the exact same drug. The only significant difference is that the maroon and red capsules are priced at $35.20 for a bottle of one hundred wholesale and the white capsules are $25.24.

Ⅰrand-name companies have developed a number of ways to deal with generic competition. Sometimes, like SmithKline Beecham, they make capsules for generic firms, which sell the drugs under the generic firm's label. Sometimes they simply package their brand-name product with a generic label of their own, charging substantially less than the brand-name version, which they continue to sell at a high price. Sometimes only the active ingredients are sold. Sometimes the generic companies sell the entire product to the brand-name companies.

Imperial Chemical Industries (ICI) used several of these strategies with its widely prescribed heart drug, Tenormin (generic name, atenolol).

First ICI set up its own generic firm in Puerto Rico, called IPR, which started manufacturing atenolol under its label. Then, in February of 1992, ICI expanded its presence in the generic market by teaming up with the major generic drug house, Goldline Labs.

Even though the atenolol being sold under the three different labels was identical—all coming off the same assembly line in Puerto Rico—the prices were not. The list price to pharmacies for a bottle of one hundred pills (50 mg), for instance, varied by more than 75 percent. ICI's brand-name version cost $80.20. IPR's atenolol cost $65.02. And Goldline Lab's atenolol cost $45.25.

Why did ICI do this? The industry publication *Pink Sheet* explained it simply: "The different marketing arms represent attempts to reach different segments of the market at different prices."

Another way drug companies keep the generics at bay is by giving the old drug a face lift, enough of an improvement to justify additional protection from the Food and Drug Administration or the Patent Office. Typically, the change involves reducing the number of times a patient needs to take the drug each day—a big selling point because it means a patient is less likely to forget to take the medicine. Sometimes the change is only significant enough to qualify for a few years of extra protection, granted by the FDA. At other times the changes are sufficient to justify a completely new seventeen-year patent.

Pfizer's hypertension drug Procardia is a good example of how drug companies do this. Pfizer came out with Procardia XL in 1989, two years before the original Procardia's patent expired. Using a complicated manufacturing process, drug makers were able to produce a pill that would slowly release its active ingredient over a twenty-four-hour period.

Procardia XL had the same active ingredients as immediate-release Procardia, but the Patent Office considered the process to produce XL novel. It granted a new patent protecting the way XL is made until 2003. This, in effect, continues the market protection for XL.

Pfizer filled medical journals with ads touting once-a-day drug schedules, and Procardia XL sold fast. The promotion people had only two years to establish physician loyalty to XL before cheaper generic copies of original Procardia came on the market.

Two years after XL's introduction, Pfizer's success was reported this way in the *F-D-C Reports* (*Pink Sheet*), a trade publication: "Sales [of Procardia XL] in 1991 were up 95 percent, more than offsetting a 67 percent decline in sales of immediate-release Procardia, which now faces generic competition."

Sometimes companies take even more drastic action to breathe new life into products that are losing patent protection. They reformulate and weaken them so the drugs can be sold over the counter. Over-the-counter drugs are a huge and growing market.

These strategic moves to counteract patent expirations may be effective in protecting company profits, but they often add to mounting drug costs. Sustained-release drugs often keep customers from going to the cheaper generic version of the original. And although the over-the-counter forms of drugs are usually cheaper than the original prescription drugs, they are rarely covered by insurance, so the consumer may end up paying more.

The pharmaceutical industry is reshaping the vistas of Barceloneta, Puerto Rico, an agricultural community west of San Juan. The pineapple fields have been crowded out by sprawling factory complexes. The old military road south of town has become a four-lane highway, busy with trucks headed to and from San Juan. Lush hillsides, rising sharply from the flatlands, have been bulldozed aside.

This community is now home to one of the thickest concentrations of drug manufacturing in the world. Along a three-mile stretch of highway are factories that produce some of the most popular prescription drugs in America, generating at least $3 billion a year in sales.

South of the road is Merck & Co., which makes the key chemical component for its blockbuster cholesterol drug, Mevacor. Nearby, Bristol-Meyers Squibb Corp. produces antibiotics, and Sterling Winthrop Inc. makes painkillers. On the north side of the highway, Abbott Laboratories churns out tranquilizers, and Pfizer Inc. pounds out its Procardia medicines for hypertension. A mile west in neighboring Arecibo is Upjohn Co., which makes two of America's best-known psycho-pharmaceutical drugs—Xanax for anxiety and Halcion for sleep.

The companies have been drawn here by huge federal tax concessions and generous local breaks. Congress passed the tax incentives to create jobs and strengthen the poor economic base of Puerto Rico, a U.S. commonwealth. About 20,000 pharmaceutical jobs have resulted.

There has been another, less visible effect. For each new job created by the drug companies with an average compensation of $26,500 a year, the companies received an annual tax break of $70,788. That's the way it is with the drug industry. The good it does for society is far more conspicuous than the good it does for itself.

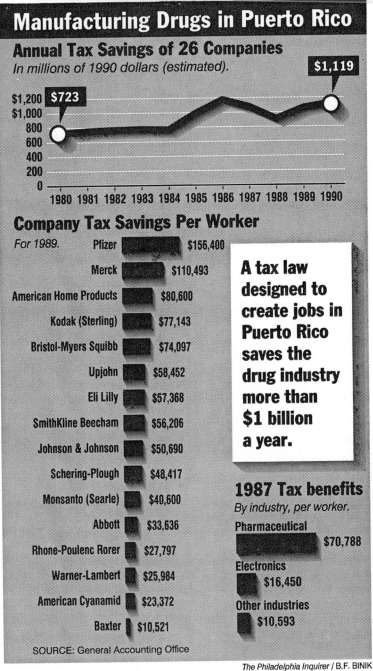

Manufacturing Drugs in Puerto Rico

Annual Tax Savings of 26 Companies
In millions of 1990 dollars (estimated).

$723

$1,119

| | 1980 | 1981 | 1982 | 1983 | 1984 | 1985 | 1986 | 1987 | 1988 | 1989 | 1990 |

($1,200, $1,000, 800, 600, 400, 200, 0)

Company Tax Savings Per Worker

For 1989.

Pfizer	$156,400
Merck	$110,493
American Home Products	$80,600
Kodak (Sterling)	$77,143
Bristol-Myers Squibb	$74,097
Upjohn	$58,452
Eli Lilly	$57,368
SmithKline Beecham	$56,206
Johnson & Johnson	$50,690
Schering-Plough	$48,417
Monsanto (Searle)	$40,600
Abbott	$33,636
Rhone-Poulenc Rorer	$27,797
Warner-Lambert	$25,984
American Cyanamid	$23,372
Baxter	$10,521

A tax law designed to create jobs in Puerto Rico saves the drug industry more than $1 billion a year.

1987 Tax benefits
By industry, per worker.

Pharmaceutical
$70,788

Electronics
$16,450

Other industries
$10,593

SOURCE: General Accounting Office

The Philadelphia Inquirer / B.F. BINIK

N

othing better illustrates the industry's profit-making ingenuity than the way the drug companies have taken advantage of Section 936 of the U.S. tax code.

Congress exempted companies that established manufacturing facilities on the island from paying federal income taxes on their Puerto Rican income. Thanks to the tax break, the twenty-six major drug companies operating in Puerto Rico make about 60 cents profit on every dollar's worth of sales—or about four times what they make on the mainland, according to the Economic Development Administration in Puerto Rico. As a result, about 20 percent of all drugs sold in the United States are now manufactured in Puerto Rico.

The tax provision, enacted in 1976, wasn't written with the drug business specifically in mind, but it has profited more than any other industry. The electronics industry, for instance, received an average tax benefit of $16,450 per Puerto Rican employee, compared to the drug companies' average of $70,788. A General Accounting Office review of 1987 statistics revealed that the drug industry received $1.3 billion, or 56 percent of all the Section 936 tax benefits that year, but it created only 18 percent of the jobs.

The reason the drug industry's per-employee, as well as total, tax savings are so much more than other industries' is that the tax break is geared to profit, not to the number of jobs created. The drug companies are not labor-intensive, but they do make a large profit, much more than other businesses. And they capitalized on their advantage by moving some of their most profitable drugs to Puerto Rico. Hence, drug companies did not create a lot of jobs on the island for the amount of tax savings they got. For every dollar in salary paid to Puerto Rican workers, the drug companies got an average of $2.67 in tax benefits.

Drug companies take advantage of the U.S. tax code in several ways. First, they deduct fully their research expenses for a drug discovered on the mainland. Then, they are able to exempt from taxes a sizable portion of a drug's income when it is produced in Puerto Rico. Johnson & Johnson profited the most from the tax law, saving an estimated $1.1 billion between 1980 and 1990 (in 1990 dollars), the GAO report showed. SmithKline Beecham saved $987 million.

The tax break is so significant that it substantially reduces the overall corporate tax rates of these companies. A 1990 Prudential Securities report said, "Puerto Rican manufacturing is the primary reason for the industry's low tax rate—28.5 percent on average." The U.S. corporate rate is 34 percent. The 936 provision will cost the Treasury $15 billion from 1993 through 1997, the Congressional Budget Office estimates.

It is "indefensible," said Sen. David Pryor (D., Ark.), chairman of the Senate Special Committee on Aging, who asked the GAO to prepare the study. "This GAO report proves we squander billions of precious tax dollars on an industry which needs little help from the federal government," Pryor said on May 14, 1992, when the report was released.

Senator William S. Cohen (R., Maine) said the Puerto Rican investment credit "has become a tax incentive that rewards the spiraling escalation of drug prices. Because this tax credit is based on profits, the higher the drug companies' prices, the greater the amount of tax credits the drug companies can claim."

The drug industry, however, is not inclined to take the blame for a situation that Congress created. "Industry did what government asked it to do in helping out the Puerto Rican economy," said Joseph Scodari, vice president and general manager of U.S. pharmaceuticals at Rhone-Poulenc Rorer. "The government put incentives in place to foster development."

"We didn't ask the federal government to put us in Puerto Rico," said Paul Freiman, chairman and chief executive officer of Syntex Corp. "They asked us to operate on the island to provide jobs. We have invested heavily and created an infrastructure that makes us competitive with the Germans and Japanese. The industry is a bit of a jewel."

The Puerto Rican tax incentive also has resulted in lost tax revenue for the places where the companies previously had their operations. American Home Products, for instance, closed its pharmaceutical plant in Elkhart, Ind., in 1991, putting eight hundred people out of work. The projected lost revenue over two years was $6.2 million in federal income tax, $1.41 million in state income tax, $220,000 in property tax, and $430,500 in sales and excise tax, according to the Midwest Center for Labor Research. Total cost to government over the two-year period: an estimated $36.7 million.

In return, Puerto Rico gets 20,000 pharmaceutical jobs and spin-off employment. The companies estimate that four local jobs are created for every Section 936 job. Even so, in Barceloneta, about 60 percent of the residents live below the poverty level. And in the midst of all this pharmaceutical activity, the health clinic still doesn't get enough medicine.

Why isn't the community benefiting more from the drug industry's presence? Manufacturing companies, including the drug firms, pay very low Puerto Rican income taxes—4.5 percent on profits, almost one tenth of the top tax rate for nonmanufacturing companies. They also get significant breaks on local business and property taxes.

The Section 936 tax break has become so controversial that Congress is considering modifying the law. In 1992, Senator Pryor tried to link the tax benefits to a requirement that price increases be held within the rate of inflation, but the bill was tabled.

"You know what happens if they pull the rug on Puerto Rico?" asked Alberto Salazar, who heads the Puerto Rican Economic Development Administration. "We will all go to the mainland on a one-way ticket."

Without 936, the drug companies also might be on the move.

"What would probably happen," said Senator Dave Durenberger (R., Minn.) during debate on the Pryor proposal, "is that the pharmaceutical companies will move their Puerto Rican processing operations to a tax-haven country like Ireland, or a low-wage developing country in the Far East."

Across the plains of North America, nearly five hundred ranchers and farmers collect the raw material for one of the most prescribed drugs in the United States. For fifty years the ritual has been the same. Every winter, they strap a diaper-like apparatus on their pregnant mares and collect the horses' urine.

Periodically a truck from Wyeth-Ayerst Laboratories picks up the urine. The company extracts and refines a hormone from it used to produce Premarin, a popular drug used to treat such postmenopausal symptoms as hot flashes.

Nothing substantially has changed in the way the drug is collected or made since Premarin's introduction into the U.S. market fifty years ago. Except the cost. Since 1985, when the company advertised Premarin as an "unparalleled value" for less than 20 cents a day, the price has risen by at least 75 percent, to thirty-five cents a day.

In the late 1970s, studies started to show that the drug helped prevent osteoporosis, the brittle bones often found in postmenopausal women. Then doctors learned in the mid-1980s that the drug also reduces a woman's chances of developing heart disease. The drug became more attractive.

The rapid price rises occurred even though Premarin was the same drug Wyeth-Ayerst had been selling for years, a drug that had long since made back its R&D cost.

"I think the Premarin pricing is incredibly low—thirty-five cents a day," said Fred Hassan, president of Wyeth-Ayerst. "If you can keep out of the hospital [by avoiding breaking a hip, for instance], the cost benefit is dramatic. It is from old drugs [like this] that we have the ability to do reseach on new drugs."

Premarin is now making more than $500 million a year in U.S. sales, making it one of the hottest selling drugs in America.

Drug companies increase the prices of their drugs not just to pay for R&D but to maintain generous profit margins. They do it on new drugs. And they do it on old drugs that have long since recouped their R&D costs.

Price Increases of Top 15 Prescribed Drugs

Average wholesale prices, from 1986 to 1991.

Product	Use	1986	1991	% Change
Amoxil (SmithKline Beecham)	infections	$21.07	$21.60	2.5%
Premarin (Wyeth Ayerst)	osteoporosis*	$15.35	$33.09	115.6%
Zantac (Glaxo)	ulcer	$60.95	$88.44	45.1%
Lanoxin (Burroughs Wellcome)	heart failure	$7.20	$9.40	30.6%
Xanax (Upjohn)	anxiety	$30.35	$59.76	96.9%
Synthroid (Boots-Flint)	thyroid	$9.13	$17.40	90.6%
Ceclor (Lilly)	infections	$111.65	$175.50	57.2%
Seldane (Marion Merrell Dow)	allergies	$48.33	$77.22	59.8%
Procardia (Pfizer)	angina	$29.50	$51.78	75.5%
Vasotec (Merck)	hypertension	$55.27	$83.63	51.3%
Cardizem (Marion Merrell Dow)	angina	$41.88	$55.08	31.5%
Tenormin (ICI)	hypertension	n/a	$77.71	n/a
Naprosyn (Syntex)	arthritis	$63.46	$86.83	36.8%
Dyazide (SmithKline Beecham)	hypertension	$22.40	$33.50	49.6%
Ortho-Novum (Ortho)	birth control	$77.10	$115.20	49.4%

SOURCE: National Association of Chain Drugstores

* Menopause

The Philadelphia Inquirer / B.F. BINIK

"The highest prescription drug price inflation occurs on drugs that have been on the market for many years, for which research-and-development costs have long since been recovered," the Senate Special Committee on Aging reported in 1991.

The report said that between 1985 and 1990:

- Synthroid, a thyroid replacement therapy made by Boots Pharmaceuticals and launched in 1938, had average annual price increases of 15.5 percent. Boots, a British firm, acquired Synthroid in 1986.
- Dilantin, an antiepileptic drug made by Parke-Davis and introduced in 1953, had annual price increases of more than 11 percent.
- Tylenol with codeine, a widely used moderate pain killer marketed by McNeil Pharmaceuticals since 1977, had a cumulative price inflation of 128.5 percent.

Even Merck & Co., one of the most innovative companies in the business, boosts the prices of its old drugs. Between 1981 and 1991, when general consumer inflation rose 50 percent, the wholesale price for a hundred-pill bottle of:

- Cogentin, a drug for Parkinson's disease, approved by the FDA in 1954, rose 208 percent, to $16.78.
- Decadron, an allergy medicine approved in 1958, rose 206 percent, to $42.50.
- Aldomet, a hypertension medicine approved in 1962, rose 168 percent, to $30.76.

These three drugs are so old that they parallel the long career of P. Roy Vagelos, Merck's chairman. When Merck started to sell Cogentin in 1954, Vagelos was a medical student at Columbia University. When Merck launched Decadron in 1958, he was celebrating his twenty-ninth birthday and his second year at the National Institutes of Health. When Aldomet reached the market in 1962, Vagelos was working as a research scientist in a biochemistry laboratory at the National Institutes of Health.

During all those years, Vagelos was steadily advancing his career, a career that ultimately would make him the highest-paid drug-company executive in 1990, when his compensation from Merck was $7.5 million. And during all those years, Merck was steadily advancing the prices of these drugs, which have long since paid off their R&D costs.

Drug companies advanced prices so aggressively in the 1980s that some drug company executives are concerned they might have overdone things. Coming under increasingly uncomfortable scrutiny by Congress since 1990, some companies have offered promises and compromises to blunt the cry for more controls.

The Pharmaceutical Manufacturers Association has made more accessible the list of free-drug programs by its members. A few firms have announced they would give public health clinics a price break on their drugs. The most dramatic of the promises has been a pledge by seven companies to keep price increases within the rate of inflation. Merck's Vagelos first made the pledge in 1990; six other companies have since followed suit.

"I think the industry has to—and has—moderated pricing," said Paul E. Freiman, chairman and chief executive officer of Syntex Corp.

But Tom Snedden, director of the subsidized prescription drug program for low-income older citizens in Pennsylvania, known as the Pharmaceutical Assistance Contract for the Elderly (PACE), said companies aren't holding the line on all drugs being sold to PACE customers. Snedden said most companies, including those that have made the pledge, are increasing prices of some medicines much faster than inflation, as measured by the Consumer Price Index.

The cost of many drugs to PACE, which pays for one out of every five prescriptions filled at drugstores in Pennsylvania, climbed faster than general inflation, even though the state was able to persuade drug companies to give PACE a 12.5-percent discount in 1991. Some significant drugs increased so much that even the discount didn't make up the difference.

The upshot? The industry recouped the rebate and pocketed an additional $4 million, Snedden said.

Schondelmeyer, the Minnesota economist, said companies restrain price increases to their most price-sensitive customers, such as hospitals and health maintenance organizations, while raising prices faster to the retail customer. The two average out, bringing them within the Consumer Price Index.

Merck has continued to raise its list prices to pharmacies on some of its top-sellers, even though it set the precedent in making the first pledge to hold down increases in the spring of 1990.

Here's what happened to prices between November 1990 and November 1992, when consumer prices rose by 6.1 percent, according to average wholesale prices supplied by the Pennsylvania PACE program:

- 10.9 percent increase on Mevacor, a cholesterol drug.
- 13.2 percent increase on Vasotec, a hypertension medicine.
- 13.2 percent increase on Pepcid, an ulcer medicine.

"It's just another indication of how the manufacturers turn you every way but loose," Snedden said. "It is another example of how difficult it is to get a break in an unregulated price environment. I really get frustrated with this. I can't think of any way, short of regulating drug prices nationally, to get programs like PACE a drug-company break on price."

Government pressure, large purchasing groups, and consumer outrage ultimately may force drug companies to show restraint in raising the prices of existing drugs, but the industry still has its mega-weapon: New drugs.

Each generation of new drugs is much more costly than the generation before it, sometimes two, three, or even ten times more expensive than the medicines they replace. The drug industry makes no bones about that. "For medicines that the company believes are clearly superior to earlier products, we do charge more," Merck's Vagelos wrote in a 1991 article that the company referred to instead of granting an interview.

Congress may figure out a way to hold down Medicaid costs, or HMOs may bargain for good deals on drugs, but the price of new drugs keeps rising. For their unique agents coming onto the market under patent protection, drug companies may charge whatever they please.

"They charge huge prices for new technologies," said Norrie Thomas, who runs a pharmacy-benefits management company in Minneapolis. "New technology is good and an American value. The thing that is wrong is that people expect health care to be responding to competitive forces, and it doesn't. If you get a new VCR, the first year it is expensive. As people keep buying them, they come down in price. That does not happen with pharmaceuticals."

There was a time when Pennsylvania Hospital would pay roughly $300 to cover two weeks of drug treatment for a typical cancer patient, said Anthony Pasquarella, director of pharmacy. No longer. Now the cancer patient often receives a new high-technology drug called Neupogen, which boosts the white-cell count depleted by the chemotherapy. The cost to the hospital for an average treatment: $1,700.

With a higher white-cell count, the patient can tolerate more chemotherapy, which he gets, sometimes doubling the original $300 treatment costs. And the nausea that accompanies chemotherapy can now be prevented with Zofran, which costs $150 per treatment. Total cost to the hospital for two weeks of chemotherapy is about $2,500—more than eight times what it used to cost. The patient's bill is even more— more than $3,000, which includes the hospital's markup.

"It keeps snowballing," Pasquarella said.

Just between 1991 and 1992, Pennsylvania Hospital's total pharmacy budget increased 20 percent. Pennsylvania Hospital is no different from all the other medical facilities, groaning under the increasing weight of new medicines with steep prices. And on the horizon, thanks to breakthroughs in biotechnology, are many more drugs that will cost thousands of dollars per treatment.

It's just the beginning.

4.
Getting around the risks of research and development

For three years, Rutgers University biochemist Abraham Abuchowski had traipsed around the country trying to persuade research directors of the nation's major drug companies that he had found a way to make cancer drugs safer and more effective.

The companies were aware of the limitations of some cancer drugs. The drugs often caused severe toxic reactions and had to be discontinued before they could do much good. Sometimes the body's immune system recognized them as foreign protein and attacked the drugs.

Abuchowski had discovered that by attaching fragments of protein called poly(ethylene) glycol (PEG) to the molecule that constitutes the cancer drug, he could prevent the destructive immune response and toxic reaction. It seemed like an important advance, but the drug companies weren't interested.

So Abuchowski formed his own company, Enzon Inc., in 1983. A year later, Enzon started trials in four hundred children with acute lymphoblastic leukemia. The company tested a modified form of asparaginase, a leukemia drug that was very effective but so toxic that it had to be discontinued in 70 percent of patients. Preliminary results with the modified drug showed that less than 3 percent of the children suffered serious negative reactions, while 70 percent showed major improvement.

Enzon's version of the drug was awaiting government approval. The first beneficiaries would be leukemia patients. But Abuchowski

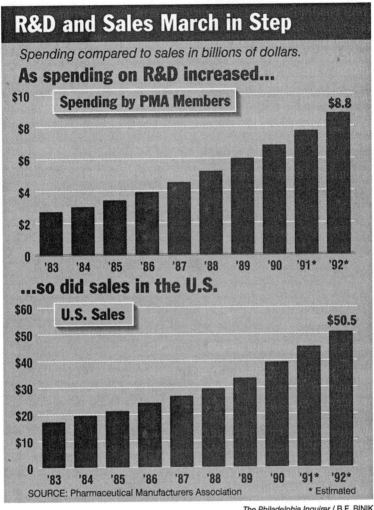

R&D and Sales March in Step

Spending compared to sales in billions of dollars.

As spending on R&D increased...

Spending by PMA Members

$8.8

'83 '84 '85 '86 '87 '88 '89 '90 '91* '92*

...so did sales in the U.S.

U.S. Sales

$50.5

'83 '84 '85 '86 '87 '88 '89 '90 '91* '92*

SOURCE: Pharmaceutical Manufacturers Association   * Estimated

The Philadelphia Inquirer / B.F. BINIK

thinks the PEG system can be extended to a host of other drugs and cancers. Are drug firms interested now?

"I think they are assessing all of this in their own methodical and careful way," Abuchowski said. "Large companies with lots of money will wait until a small company gets far enough along. They will wait until it's a sure thing, and then buy the idea or the company itself. It makes good business sense."

Whenever drug industry executives are challenged at congressional hearings by legislators looking into the high cost of drugs, their response is the same: Pharmaceutical research is very expensive. It costs an average of $231 million for each drug brought to market. Sixteen cents of every sales dollar is spent on drug R&D, three times the average for other industries. For every discovery that results in a breakthrough drug, many expensive efforts fail.

To hear drug companies tell it, this must be a very difficult business in which to survive. Yet they not only survive, they manage to absorb all these costs and remain the most profitable businesses in America. That's because drug companies—especially the big brand-name ones, which account for the majority of drug research—are able to minimize their R&D risks in many ways:

- They make "me-too" drugs, duplicating medicines that are already proven successes.
- They buy other people's research or merge with companies that have promising drugs.
- They benefit from basic research done by federal and academic laboratories.
- They get substantial tax breaks or other incentives to develop and produce many of the drugs for which they charge high prices.
- They abandon research on potentially useful drugs when market analysis shows the expected profit is not going to be big enough.
- They even put premium prices on drugs they did not develop.

Letting someone else do the basic or preliminary research until a project looks as if it will pay off handsomely is one of the surest ways the big companies have of minimizing risk. This is what they are doing with Abuchowski. Once a company does decide to develop or build on someone else's discovery, it often puts a high price on the drug, even though little of the company's own money was spent on the preliminary research.

That's what Wyeth-Ayerst Laboratories did with the contraceptive Norplant. It's what Janssen Pharmaceutica Inc. did with a cancer drug called levamisole. And it's what Burroughs Wellcome Co. did with AZT, the first drug effective in slowing the development of AIDS.

The research people at Wyeth-Ayerst, which sells Norplant in this country, had little interest in the idea of a long-acting contraceptive when it was first proposed to them years ago. Wyeth was one of several big firms that rejected the idea when the nonprofit Population Council of New York City tried to interest them in it, a research scientist at the council said.

So with funding from the Rockefeller and Ford foundations and the Agency for International Development, the council went ahead on its

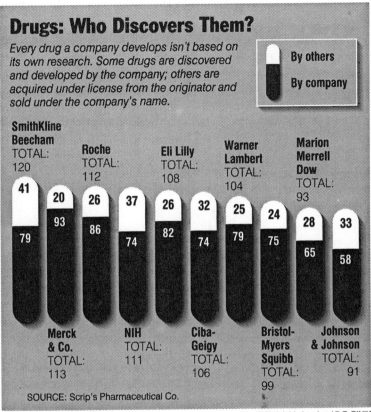

Drugs: Who Discovers Them?

Every drug a company develops isn't based on its own research. Some drugs are discovered and developed by the company; others are acquired under license from the originator and sold under the company's name.

By others

By company

SmithKline Beecham TOTAL: 120 — 41 / 79

Roche TOTAL: 112 — 20 / 93

Eli Lilly TOTAL: 108 — 26 / 86

Warner Lambert TOTAL: 104 — 37 / 74

Marion Merrell Dow TOTAL: 93 — 26 / 82

Merck & Co. TOTAL: 113 — 32 / 74

NIH TOTAL: 111 — 25 / 79

Ciba-Geigy TOTAL: 106 — 24 / 75

Bristol-Myers Squibb TOTAL: 99 — 28 / 65

Johnson & Johnson TOTAL: 91 — 33 / 58

SOURCE: Scrip's Pharmaceutical Co.

The Philadelphia Inquirer / B.F. BINIK

own, said Irving Sivin, a senior associate and biostatistician with the Population Council. The council spent $10 million and several years running clinical trials with the matchstick-thin Norplant capsules, which are implanted under the skin and slowly release the hormone progestin.

Though Wyeth chose not to do the R&D, the company did want to stay on top of the research. So Wyeth provided the Population Council free of charge the hormone progestin, which it had developed, for use in the trials, with the provision that it would have first rights to distribute the drug in the United States should the trials prove successful.

The trials did prove Norplant's success. Wyeth still wasn't interested in risking capital in the manufacture of the contraceptive. So the Population Council turned to the Finnish firm of Leiras Pharmaceutical, which decided to make the drug.

Wyeth subsequently activated its right to distribute the contraceptive in the United States, paying a royalty to the Population Council. Buying Norplant from Leiras, it repackages the contraceptive and sells it for $365—almost four times as much as the $96 that Finnish women pay for the drug. Americans have to pay this premium even though Norplant was developed with U.S. government and philanthropic funds.

Sandra Waldman, a spokeswoman for the Population Council, said attempts were made to persuade Wyeth to sell Norplant to public agencies at a lower price.

Wyeth spokeswoman Audrey Ashby said the company didn't get involved with Norplant's R&D because "preliminary research showed that it would not be accepted by American women. We did not want to have a brand new contraceptive for American women that would not succeed."

Norplant is turning out to be a very important contraceptive.

Asked why Norplant costs so much more in the United States, Ashby said Wyeth spent $30 million to train 30,000 doctors in inserting and removing Norplant. And Wyeth includes the tools needed for these procedures as part of the drug's purchase price, she said.

Sometimes it is research done by academic physicians that drug companies profit from. These are the doctors who independently run lengthy trials showing how a drug being sold for one medical problem can be used effectively for a different one.

Janssen Pharmaceutica benefited in this way with levamisole, a veterinary drug it discovered that turned out to be very effective against cancer in humans.

For years levamisole had been used to rid sheep of parasites. Because the drug also seemed to improve animals' immune systems, doctors such as Charles G. Moertel of the Mayo Comprehensive Cancer Center started testing the drug in human cancer patients in 1978. Supported with $11 million in grants from the National Cancer Institute, Moertel studied the drug with 1,300 colon cancer patients. In 1992, Moertel reported the results of the ongoing trials: He was able to cut the death rate by a third and the recurrence of cancer by 40 percent, using levamisole in conjunction with another cancer drug.

Moertel said in a recent interview that Janssen, a subsidiary of Johnson & Johnson, had promised him and other researchers that the drug for human use, to be called Ergamisol, would be sold at a reasonable price.

A year's supply of Ergamisol costs $1,250 to $1,500. The same amounts purchased at the price of the sheep drug would cost $14, Moertel said. Why such a large difference?

"We think the price is reasonable," said Robert Kniffen, spokesman for Janssen Pharmaceutica Inc. "You are talking about a drug for someone with colon cancer who goes on the drug for a year. . . . On average it costs something like $1,300 a year, which is the cost of one day in the hospital. Here is a therapy that helps and saves and prolongs people's lives."

Sometimes it is the government that does work that drug companies profit from.

Burroughs Wellcome Co. has the U.S. government to thank for the fortune it made from zidovudine (AZT), the first drug for AIDS.

AZT, brand-name Retrovir, had been synthesized as a cancer drug in 1964 by a government-funded scientist in Detroit. But it wasn't effective against cancer and was forgotten for more than a decade until Burroughs Wellcome Co. took it up with the intention of developing AZT as an antibacterial. The company ultimately decided against that.

It wasn't until several years later, after the first AIDS cases were recognized in 1981, that AZT resurfaced, this time in a National Cancer Institute laboratory. In response to appeals from the institute, drug companies had been supplying compounds that might be effective against the newly discovered AIDS virus, and Burroughs Wellcome had sent AZT to be tested. Not only did AZT prove to be effective in laboratory studies, in subsequent trials it slowed progression of the disease in humans.

All this tax-supported assistance and encouragement didn't stop Burroughs Wellcome from setting the initial price for AZT treatment at $10,000 a year. Following a rash of protests and demonstrations by AIDS victims, the company dropped the price by 20 percent in December 1987, less than a year after it came on the market.

The riskiest and most costly research is the very basic research that has no clear-cut applications. It is the fundamental research that leads to the discoveries that win Nobel Prizes. This is the research that often begins with childlike questions: Why is the sky blue? Why are roses red? Why do hearts beat? Why do cancer cells keep multiplying?

It's the answers to such basic questions that can lead to a myriad of new drugs. Commercially motivated drug companies rarely can afford the luxury of asking them, though, because no one can predict if, let alone when, the answers will come.

"A company won't get involved if the expectation is that the research won't pay off for ten years," said Ralph F. Hirschmann, a research professor of chemistry at the University of Pennsylvania and a former senior vice president for basic research at Merck & Co. "The trick of being a good research director is recognizing when research has reached the point that it can be exploited within five years."

That's why drug companies rely heavily on tax-supported academia and the National Institutes of Health, which focuses on basic research. That also helps to explain why seventy-four NIH-supported scientists went on to win the Nobel Prize, compared to three from drug companies, even though the industry spends more on R&D than the National Institutes of Health.

Government scientists at the National Institutes of Health want to see practical applications come from their work and have provided their findings and research free to industry. Scientists have expressed concern, though, over the high prices companies have set for such drugs as Retrovir.

Recently government laboratories have begun to establish contractual relationships with private industry, which will support scientific projects or scientists the companies are interested in. The Federal Technology Transfer Act, passed in 1986, encourages the transfer of knowledge to private industry. These contracts, called collaborative research and development agreements (CRADAs), contain provisions that products developed from this joint research will be priced reasonably. The provision has been in effect since 1989.

Drug company involvement with outside laboratories is likely to grow in coming years.

A 1991 study cited by the federal Office of Technology Assessment found that by contributing a relatively small amount to the projects of academic researchers, the drug firms gain "access to research, expertise, and skill developed with public funds." Twenty-five percent of drugs produced by the pharmaceutical industry, the study said, could not have been developed without substantial delay or cost in the absence of academic research.

The government report, which has not yet been published, criticized government agencies for not being more effective in forcing fair prices. "The NIH and other federal research programs do not adequately protect the public's investment in drug discovery, development, and evaluation. These agencies lack expertise . . . in negotiating limits on prices to be charged for drugs discovered or developed with federal funds."

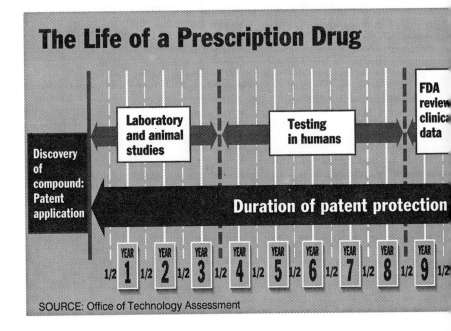

The Life of a Prescription Drug

Discovery of compound: Patent application

Laboratory and animal studies

Testing in humans

FDA review clinical data

Duration of patent protection

YEAR 1/2 1 1/2 2 1/2 3 1/2 4 1/2 5 1/2 6 1/2 7 1/2 8 1/2 9 1/2

SOURCE: Office of Technology Assessment

Although the big drug companies get a lot of research help from outside sources, the bulk of the development work is done by their own highly paid scientists. The goal is not just to find useful drugs, but to find drugs that will be profitable.

Driven by the need to generate quarterly earnings for investors, major drug companies focus R&D efforts on developing potential blockbusters—drugs that bring in $500 million a year or more in worldwide sales. This kind of research is very costly, but there are ways to minimize the risk. The most effective way is simply to duplicate existing treatments.

Fifty-three percent of the 258 drugs approved in the United States during the decade ending in 1991 were "me-too" drugs. They were classified by the Food and Drug Administration as 1C drugs, meaning they offered little or no therapeutic gain over existing remedies. Only 16 percent of the drugs were classified 1A, meaning they represented significant improvements over drugs already on the market. Trying to make better versions of existing drugs is appealing to a pharmaceutical company because the original drug's success proves the existence of a profitable market. Also, it proves that such a drug can be made.

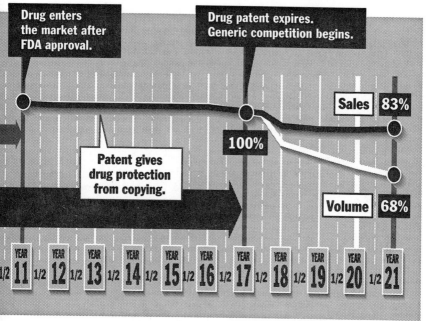

Drug enters the market after FDA approval.

Drug patent expires. Generic competition begins.

Patent gives drug protection from copying.

Sales 83%

100%

Volume 68%

YEAR 1/2 11 1/2 YEAR 12 1/2 YEAR 13 1/2 YEAR 14 1/2 YEAR 15 1/2 YEAR 16 1/2 YEAR 17 1/2 YEAR 18 1/2 YEAR 19 1/2 YEAR 20 1/2 YEAR 21

The Philadelphia Inquirer / B.F. BINIK

"As soon as a successful new drug appears on the market, its producer can be certain that competing companies are likely to soon have fifteen or more similar products in the testing phase . . ." a report issued in 1991 by the U.S. International Trade Commission said. "Even a less effective me-too drug can do well in the market, depending on the way it's promoted."

Me-too drugs come about in all sorts of ways. Sometimes companies make a few changes in the molecular structure of a successful drug to get around the patent of a competitor. At other times several companies simultaneously try to exploit the same basic research breakthrough and understandably end up with similar drugs.

It's almost like many locksmiths designing keys for the same lock. Though the keys may be made from different materials and have different designs, they can open only one lock. And in the pharmaceutical industry, when one company finds a key to a lock that's never been opened before, the others want their own keys.

That's what happened in 1976 when SmithKline Corp., now SmithKline Beecham, introduced Tagamet on the British market. It reached the U.S. market a year later.

Everyone in the industry knew SmithKline had a big winner. The drug cleared up gastric ulcers in a few weeks or months of treatment and saved thousands of patients from diets and surgical treatments that were not very effective. Truly a major success story for the pharmaceutical industry, the drug was based on a breakthrough discovery by SmithKline researcher Sir James Black. (The British scientist was knighted and awarded a Nobel Prize for this and other pioneering work.)

Black discovered a new class of cellular receptors, called H-2 receptors, that promote stomach acid secretion. Then he found a compound that blocked the receptors and thus ulcer-causing acid production. The compound was cimetidine (trade name, Tagamet).

Other companies couldn't make a drug identical to cimetidine because SmithKline had patented it, but they could look for another compound to block H-2 receptors. Within six years of Tagamet's approval, Glaxo Holdings came out with its ulcer drug, Zantac. Within eleven years, two more companies were selling H-2 receptor antagonists.

This follow-the-leader strategy is not unusual. In another scientific breakthrough, Black discovered that by blocking another group of receptors associated with heart activity, it was possible to control blood pressure and prevent angina, a type of chest pain associated with heart disease. The revolutionary new drug was called a beta-adrenergic blocker, because this was the type of receptor it blocked. The drug was approved for marketing in the United States in 1967. There are now no fewer than a dozen beta blockers on the market.

Cardiology is a Mecca for me-too drugs. Not only is heart disease the biggest killer in the western world, but its victims must take drugs for life.

"Currently, we believe that there are well over thirty-three antihypertensive agents at various stages of development," said financial analyst Hemant K. Shah.

Heart disease has made a lot of money for the pharmaceutical industry, with worldwide sales of cardiovascular drugs estimated at $22 billion in 1990. For heart patients on drugs to control cholesterol, blood pressure, and heart activity, an annual drug bill of $1,000 is common.

Because heart patients may live another thirty years after the first symptoms appear and often must take drugs for life, getting a patient on drugs is "like an annuity," said Christina Heuer, a financial analyst with Smith Barney, Harris Upham & Co.

Other specialties also have their share of me-toos. Analyst Shah said sixteen new all-purpose oral antibiotics are being developed and launched in world markets. And "we believe that due to the very successful launch of Prozac, the industry has about twenty-seven antidepressant agents in various stages of development," he said. "They all say they would like to cut back on me-too drugs, but they are not doing it."

Being neither very small nor very large, Zantac is not a very distinctive pill. Manufactured by Glaxo Holdings, it could easily be confused for aspirin, except for the words "Glaxo" and "ZANTAC" stamped into its sides.

But this is a special pill. Zantac is the biggest money-making drug in the history of the pharmaceutical business. Worldwide sales of this anti-ulcer medicine were $3 billion in 1991. The market for this one pill is four times the entire budget of the Food and Drug Administration—almost thirteen times more than the $231 million the Pharmaceutical Manufacturers Association says it costs to bring the average drug to market. And Zantac is a me-too drug. It works on the same principle as Tagamet, which came out six years earlier and is also a billion-dollar-a-year drug.

This is a powerful object lesson for the CEO of a drug company debating whether to spend research money on looking for a drug to treat a rare disease or to go for another me-too drug.

Many times a drug company ends up with a me-too drug, not significantly better than one already on the market, simply because a competitor was first to get Food and Drug Administration approval. Having spent many millions of dollars on the research, a company will decide to spend a little more to finish its research and at least get something on the market to help pay for the R&D investment. In many cases, the market is so vast—as in the case of ulcer drugs—that it can support another drug, even though it may be no better than what's already being used.

Sometimes companies drop promising research on a unique drug, if market research suggests it won't generate a big enough profit. Large companies abandon "many products whose potential looks limited to $75–130 million," writes Jeffrey J. Kraws, a financial analyst with Alex. Brown & Sons. "When it is discovered that the compound may work, but not for a $600 million market but rather for a $75 million application, the company has to make a decision, as it is not really economically feasible to complete testing and launch the product."

That doesn't necessarily mean the idea dies, though. Roberts Pharmaceuticals is a firm that hopes to live off the crumbs from the big companies' table by taking on these abandoned drugs and developing them into profitable medicines. Roberts, for example, has been working on a drug for thrombocytosis, a blood disorder for which there is no other approved drug treatment.

Russell C. McLauchlan, president and chief operating officer of U.S.

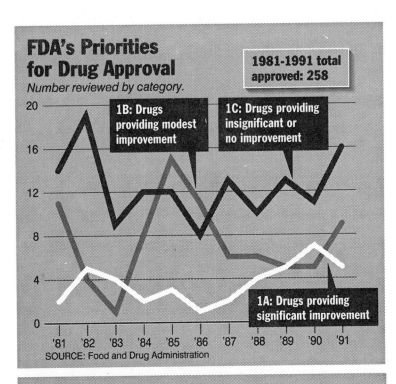

FDA's Priorities for Drug Approval

Number reviewed by category.

1981-1991 total approved: 258

- **1B: Drugs providing modest improvement**
- **1C: Drugs providing insignificant or no improvement**
- **1A: Drugs providing significant improvement**

'81 '82 '83 '84 '85 '86 '87 '88 '89 '90 '91

SOURCE: Food and Drug Administration

The Billion-Dollar Drugs

Drug name in U.S.	Originator	Condition	World sales In billions
Zantac	Glaxo Holdings Plc.	ulcer	$3.0
Procardia/Adalat	Bayer A.G.	heart	$1.9
Vasotec	Merck & Co.	heart	$1.7
Capoten	Bristol-Myers Squibb Corp.	heart	$1.6
Epogen	Amgen	acute anemia	$1.5
Ventolin/Proventil	Glaxo Holdings Plc.	asthma	$1.2
Ceclor	Eli Lilly & Co.	infections	$1.2
Cardizem	Tanabe	heart	$1.2
Mevacor	Merck & Co.	cholesterol	$1.1
Voltaren	Ciba-Geigy Ltd.	arthritis	$1.1
Zovirax	Burroughs-Wellcome	herpes	$1.1
Tenormin	ICI	heart	$1.1
Tagamet	SmithKline Beecham Plc.	ulcers	$1.0
Cipro	Bayer A.G.	infections	$1.0

SOURCE: Mehta & Isaly

The Philadelphia Inquirer / B.F. BINIK

Bioscience Inc. and formerly a vice president of Lederle Labs, says that opportunities are probably being missed all the time. He is convinced enough of this that he expects his company to make a handsome profit by taking on abandoned cancer-drug projects and developing them into successful drugs.

T he doctor didn't think that Mary Escarcega's baby girl, Mallory, would live for more than a few days. Only six weeks old, the emaciated little baby had huge eyes with a hollow, distant look. Her stomach was distended, and she labored to drink the infant formula her mother offered her as they waited in the doctor's office in Fresno, Calif.

Suspecting a rare brain disorder, the neurologist left the room in a last-ditch effort to find another reason for Mallory's condition. Ten minutes later, the doctor returned, picked up the frail infant, and took the child and her parents to yet another specialist in the hospital.

This time, the diagnosis was different. This time, the doctors said it was a rare protein deficiency, called methylmalonic acidemia. And this time there was a treatment, a drug called Carnitor made by Sigma-Tau Pharmaceuticals Inc.

Literally overnight, Mallory started to thrive. Within four days, she had gained about half a pound. Six years later, in 1992, Mallory was in first grade, healthy and happy. Mallory is alive today because a pharmaceutical company decided to make a drug even though it had little chance of becoming a blockbuster.

I t is difficult, if not impossible, to say how many more effective drugs would be available if the major companies weren't so focused on finding blockbuster drugs. But in 1983, the federal government inadvertently did an experiment that showed how the industry can do a lot more when sufficiently motivated.

The experiment was the Orphan Drug Act, which gave drug companies exclusive sales rights and tax incentives for developing drugs for rare diseases, defined by the law as those diseases affecting fewer than 200,000 Americans. It's because of this law, a Sigma-Tau representative said, that the company developed Carnitor, the drug that saved Mallory Escarcega's life.

During the decade preceding the 1983 passage of the act, the drug industry had developed ten drugs for rare diseases. Since 1983, more than six times that number have been developed. Sixty-four orphan drugs effective against sixty-seven diseases have been approved by the Food and Drug Administration, and another 314 medicines are in development as designated orphans by the agency, as of fall 1992. (The Pharmaceutical Manufacturers Association said in 1992 that its members were involved in the development of eighty-five orphan drugs.) And some of the drugs being developed are for more than one illness. Since the law was passed, drugs for 501 conditions have received Orphan Drug designation.

And what are some of these "rare" diseases that stand to benefit from this law? Leukemia. Botulism. Sickle cell anemia. Hemophilia. Multiple sclerosis. Muscular dystrophy. Cerebral palsy. Cystic fibrosis. Some forms of epilepsy. And even many infections associated with AIDS. The law "has been more successful than we could have ever imagined," said Abbey Meyers, executive director of the National Association for Rare Disorders, who lobbied for it.

In fact, many of the important drugs approved by the FDA during the last five years were orphan drugs. These were the new drugs the FDA classified as 1A because they appeared to offer "an important therapeutic gain" over existing medicines and therefore were entitled to more expeditious review.

(The agency discontinued the "1A-1B-1C" classification system in 1992, after complaints from the drug industry, an agency spokesman said. "The firms didn't like to be in the 'C' category," the spokesman, Mike Shaffer, said. "It might put them in a marketing disadvantage." The "1C" category classified a drug as offering little or no therapeutic gain. The new system has only two main classifications—one for significant new drugs and the other for the rest.

The Food and Drug Administration's system "was misunderstood, misrepresented, and misused for years, and to put it into well-deserved oblivion was a PMA priority for a very long time," John R. Stafford, chairman and chief executive officer of American Home Products, told executives at the PMA's annual convention in May 1992. "Now it is accomplished.")

Talhe future of the pharmaceutical industry may be revolutionized by biotechnology, an emerging field in which the major drug companies initially showed little interest. Having developed rapidly over the last twenty years, biotechnology uses completely different methods in discovering drugs. Whereas traditional pharmaceutical research seeks new drugs by screening thousands of compounds found in nature, biotechnology does it by reproducing the complex, naturally occurring substances in the body. Primary targets of biotechnology are such things as disease-fighting white blood cells, enzymes, hormones, and other biochemicals that play a vital role in helping living organisms function.

The development of biotechnology was spearheaded by government researchers, academic scientists, and small companies, often formed around a single scientist, working with venture capital. "The large companies sit back and wait and acquire products via small companies," said David Martin, executive vice president of research and development for Du Pont Merck Pharmaceutical Co. in Wilmington, Del. "A big company will watch a technology and see if it works. It may experiment with it. A small company will put all their eggs in one basket. The risk profile of an entrepreneur in a start-up company is much different than funding a big company."

The big companies were particularly skeptical about gene therapy, in which diseases are treated by replacing or deactivating genes that are not doing what they're supposed to be doing. "Most people viewed this as the stuff Buck Rogers is made of until the last year or two," said Marc Schneebaum, chief financial officer of Genetic Therapy Inc. of Gaithersburg, Md., a biotech firm with $40 million in assets that was started in 1986. "Virtually all the big companies are public companies, and people don't want to invest in big risks."

One reason the drug industry was at first so skeptical of biotechnology was because it uses large proteins, which are destroyed in the stomach and have to be given by injection, a very unattractive prospect for chronic patients who have to take drugs daily for life. Another reason is that it's risky to start work in a new field, where a company has little experience or expertise.

Letting smaller companies take the pioneering lead is a way to "manage risk," said Fred Hassan, president of Wyeth-Ayerth Laboratories. "It is so difficult to be a specialist in every area. Sometimes, it is better to access the specialization somewhere else."

Biotechnology has scored several successes in recent years. It has led to the development of quick tests for pregnancy, cancer, and AIDS. It has been used to produce a hepatitis vaccine, a drug that forces the bodies of anemic patients to start making red blood cells again, and a drug that shuts off heart attacks.

Encouraged by these successes, drug companies are now building up their own in-house expertise. And what they aren't developing themselves, they are acquiring through cooperative agreements with smaller companies. Biotechnology has clearly become a less risky investment.

With the drug industry's emphasis on blockbusters, a lot of other things don't get done. Three large patient populations that could benefit from more of the industry's R&D dollars are children, old people, and those hooked on drugs and alcohol.

Drug companies do not routinely test drugs in the very young or the elderly, even though these people seem to process drugs differently than middle-age adults, on whom most trials are conducted. Without trial data, physicians frequently are forced to guess at the appropriate drug dose for their young and old patients.

Seventy percent of the drugs prescribed in children's hospitals have not been approved specifically for pediatric use, said Ralph E. Kauffman of the American Academy of Pediatrics. Choosing the right dose, he said, often "ends up being an experiment in every child." It is much more complicated than simply cutting the FDA-approved adult dose in half because the child is half the size of a grown-up. The growing bodies of children handle drugs differently, he said.

Doctors treating older patients have similar problems. Adverse interactions among the many drugs older people take is a common reason for their hospitalization.

Risa J. Lavizzo-Mourey, associate professor of geriatric medicine at the University of Pennsylvania Medical Center, said it's "absolutely essential" to get more information on the best way to prescribe drugs in the elderly. By this she meant the growing population of people over seventy-five, an age when the cumulative effects of aging start changing the ways a patient's body handles drugs. She said slight differences in the response of a younger person to different drugs are greatly magnified in these older people. For instance, a drug that makes a young person slightly drowsy may make a very old person so sleepy that it's almost impossible to rouse them.

Because not enough data are available to guide physicians in prescribing for the very old, the motto is "start low and go slow," said Stanley L. Slater, deputy associate director for geriatrics at the National Institute of Aging. It is much more difficult and expensive to do studies with the very old, he said. Large numbers of test subjects are needed because old people often have a variety of diseases that confuse the results of the trials, and many drop out or die before the lengthy studies can be completed.

Slater agrees with Lavizzo-Mourey on the need for drug trials in the elderly but said he can understand why drug companies would not want to go to the trouble or expense of doing them. He sees it as a "dispute among people of good will," but still he would like to see the trials done.

The lack of clinical data on very old patients is a particular problem for cardiologists, since heart disease primarily afflicts the elderly. Yet 60 percent of the 214 heart-drug studies conducted in the last three decades excluded patients over 75, Harvard University researcher Jerry H. Gurwitz reported in September 1991. "Exclusion of the elderly prevents collection of the very data clinicians and researchers need to make informed decisions when treating this important population," Gurwitz wrote.

In October 1992, the Food and Drug Administration encouraged pharmaceutical companies to consider children when compiling data on drugs that might have pediatric uses. The agency said it would approve pediatric labeling of drugs tested exclusively in adults only if the drug companies also compiled data showing that the drug would have the same effects and be just as safe in children.

Fred Telling, a vice president for Pfizer Inc., said one reason for the industry's reluctance to do drug trials in these age groups is that companies don't want to put children and old people at risk. "The primary emphasis has to be on doing no harm to the patient," Telling said. "The older you get or the younger you are, the greater is the likelihood of an untoward effect."

Addiction to street drugs like heroin and cocaine is another growing medical problem that is wanting for lack of effective drugs. Though the need for anti-addiction medicines has been well documented for four decades, only two medicines have been developed to help heroin addicts, which total about 500,000 people in the United States. No medicine to combat cocaine addiction has yet been approved by the FDA.

"It is an unmet medical need [that] . . . has not been a high priority of the pharmaceutical industry," said Charles Grudzinskas, an official with the National Institute on Drug Abuse.

The institute has prodded a number of companies to become more involved, asking them to look for promising drugs among compounds they have already developed. A few companies have set up small research programs, said Grudzinskas. Still, he said, their efforts on substance abuse have been modest compared to their quest for other central nervous system medications, where the chance for commercial success is well established.

No medical procedure is as cost-effective or medically effective as vaccines. But only a handful of drug companies are interested in working on them. Merck & Co. is the notable exception, having maintained a strong vaccine program for years. And in 1992, SmithKline said it was expanding its vaccine business.

Other companies avoid vaccine production because the profits are low compared to other medicines, said Dr. Anthony Robbins, an expert on international vaccination efforts and a professor at the Boston University School of Public Health. According to Robbins, the combined sales of all vaccines in the world don't equal the sales of one blockbuster ulcer drug, Zantac—$3 billion. It's all very ironic, he said. Drug companies can make more money from drugs that keep alive the terminally ill "on the threshold of death" than from a low-cost vaccine for a child "on the threshold of life."

Five million to six million children in poor countries could be saved if vaccines were improved, according to the Children's Vaccine Initiative, a group formed by international relief agencies to promote vaccine development for poor countries. Economically poor nations must have vaccines that don't require refrigeration or booster shots because it is hard for families living miles from treatment sites to make the trip, often on foot, for repeat treatments. But the commerical priority for new and improved vaccines is low, Robbins said, because profit motives "guide" manufacturers to expensive vaccines in the high-priced markets of industrialized countries.

Third World countries have little money to buy drugs but have a lot of sick people who could benefit from them.

The problem is graphically illustrated in the cluttered first-floor office of Dr. Stephen L. Hoffman in the Naval Medical Research Institute Annex in Rockville, Md. In one of his two computers, Hoffman keeps a color-coded map, which uses yellow and red to represent malaria-infected areas of the world. At least one-third of the world's land mass is shaded in yellow and red. It represents an estimated 300 million infected people. Two million of them will die this year. None of the world's industrialized powers was in yellow or red.

With drug-resistant forms of the disease-carrying mosquito appearing increasingly more often, Hoffman isn't too optimistic about the prospects of new drugs that will stay ahead of the parasite. The Institute of Medicine studied the problem and concluded that the infected countries were too poor to provide the funds. The United States allocated only $31 million in 1990 for all malaria research, a fraction of what is spent on developing one drug. The drug industry isn't spending much on the problem either.

A 1990 report by the Commission on Health Research and Development said that less than 3 percent of the world pharmaceutical industry's R&D budget was directed at the health problems of poor countries. With 4.5 billion people, the Third World comprises 75 percent of the globe's population.

The one hundred companies represented by the Pharmaceutical Manufacturers Association—among the biggest and most successful firms in the world—said they would spend $10.9 billion on research and development in 1992. That's $1 billion more than the entire budget for the National Institutes of Health, the federal government's primary biomedical research effort. And it is a big share of the world's R&D. Most of the $10.9 billion will be spent by the 15 largest firms. This means that a handful of corporate executives ultimately decide which research discoveries made by the world's scientific community will reach the bedside in the form of useful medicines.

Drug company executives point out that the industry has developed scores of drugs that have substantially improved the welfare of mankind, even though more than half of the drugs approved during the last decade were considered me-too drugs. Drug companies defend the me-too drugs they are churning out, saying that the marginal advantages of these drugs are medically important and worth the cost. Because of these differences, they say, one patient may do better on one drug than another.

"None of us starts out to make a me-too drug that has no advantage," said Joseph A. Mollica, president and chief executive officer of Du Pont Merck Pharmaceutical Co. "Given the cost of research, you are not going to make your money back.

"Most of science and medicine tends to move in incremental advances," he said, citing as an example the improvements made in James Black's initial beta blocker discovery. When the first beta blocker was marketed years ago, he said, it had many side effects and had to be taken several times a day. Over the years, several types of beta blockers were discovered. Some had fewer side effects and others had to be taken less often. Now there are beta blockers that have hardly any side effects and have to be taken only once a day.

Litigation, more than anything else, is why drug companies aren't more interested in developing vaccines, company officials say. "The liability laws are incredible compared to any other country in the world," said Hassan of Wyeth-Ayerst. "The companies were driven out of the business. There was an incredible amount of litigation."

Drug company executives don't think it's necessary to defend the high profits they are making. Profit is the name of the game. Industry spokespeople say that they are in the business of making medicine and making money and that it is for society to decide, through its government, what social needs should be met. If society wants drugs for rare diseases or vaccines for public health programs or medicine for Third World countries, then it is for society to find a way to pay for this work. People should not expect a private industry to do it for them.

Philip K. Russell, professor of international health at Johns Hopkins University, sums it up: "It is incumbent on society to change the focus and not put it on the board of directors of big companies. . . . I don't think we get anything from beating up on the industry. What we need to do as a society is to perhaps change market forces."

5.
How other nations hold down drug costs

Two or three times a week, government officials gather in an office high above the Paris streets and make decisions that no public authority in the United States has the power to make. They decide the prices companies may charge for prescription drugs.

With the historic dome of the *Invalides* in the distance, they sit at a conference table and set the prices, with little concern for how much companies spent on research and development, or what size profits they say are needed to support a high-risk business, or any of the other reasons the drug industry cites for higher prices. The officials are more concerned with what impact prices will have on taxpaying voters and the French health care system, which pays most of the nation's drug bill.

Instead of debating the intricacies of pharmaceutical economics, the officials merely review prices other European nations are paying for the drug in question and then set the French price a little bit lower. Once set, the price is rarely raised significantly. It's a simple but effective system. French drug prices are among the lowest in Europe. They're 60 percent to 70 percent cheaper than prices in the United States.

Though more tightfisted than most, France is not the only country in Europe that controls drug prices. Virtually all of them do. The United States is one of very few industrialized nations in the world that do nothing to control the cost of prescription drugs. So Americans routinely pay higher prices for drugs than people in other countries.

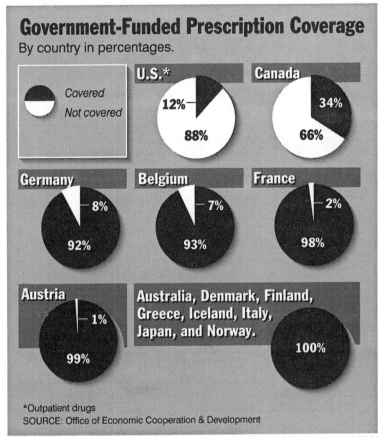

Government-Funded Prescription Coverage
By country in percentages.

- ● Covered
- ○ Not covered

U.S.* 12% — 88%

Canada 34% — 66%

Germany 8% — 92%

Belgium 7% — 93%

France 2% — 98%

Austria 1% — 99%

Australia, Denmark, Finland, Greece, Iceland, Italy, Japan, and Norway. 100%

*Outpatient drugs
SOURCE: Office of Economic Cooperation & Development

The Philadelphia Inquirer / B.F. BINIK

Each nation has its own approach.

The United Kingdom negotiates with individual companies and limits the profit each may make from selling drugs to the National Health Service, which pays for most drugs used in Britain. Once a price has been set, it is rarely raised. So the price for older drugs in Britain is far lower than comparable products in the United States, where prices are continually increasing. One study showed that drugs in the United States cost an average of 80 percent more than in the United Kingdom.

Norway won't approve a new drug unless it is cheaper or therapeutically superior to drugs already on the market.

In Canada, the Patent Medicine Prices Review Board has the power to remove patent protection from drugs it considers too costly. Largely as a result of government control, wholesale prices in Canada average 30 percent below those in the United States.

Australia, which has some of the lowest drug prices in the world, allows manufacturers to charge whatever they want, but the government sets the price the national insurance plan will pay for each drug. This price is far below what the manufacturers prefer to charge. But since the government is the primary purchaser of drugs in Australia, the companies cooperate. One study showed U.S. drug prices on average were 225 percent above those in Australia.

The Japanese government determines which drugs are covered by the nation's insurance companies and how much they will pay. Japanese prices are higher on average than European drug prices but lower than in the United States.

Some countries, such as Britain and Germany, also monitor prescribing habits of physicians and send warning letters or "advisers" to talk to those who prescribe too many or too costly drugs.

No two countries agree on the best way to do it. But, unlike the United States, they do something.

What determines whether drug prices will be high or low is government controls. Countries with strict controls have low prices. Countries with weak or no controls have high prices. This was demonstrated in 1991 in a study of one hundred of the most frequently prescribed drugs in Germany, Britain, Italy, France, Japan, and the United States. The study, by the investment firm of Lehman Bros. International, showed that the United States, with the fewest controls, had the highest prices. France, with the most restrictive controls, had the lowest.

It wasn't a fluke. The same results had been shown three years earlier in a study by the Belgian Consumers' Association, an independent not-for-profit institute similar to the Consumers Union in the United States. The study by medical sociologists Guido Adriaenssens and Guy Sermeus found that prices in Germany, the Netherlands, and Denmark, with few controls, were two to three times higher than the prices for comparable drugs in tightly regulated France, Greece, Spain, and Portugal. Some countries hold down prices so much that drug prices increase more slowly than prices of other items in the economy, the study found. The opposite is true in countries with fewer controls.

The Belgian study did not consider U.S. prices. But the staff of Sen. David Pryor of Arkansas was so intrigued by the findings that they asked Adriaenssens and Sermeus to do another survey comparing U.S. and European prices.

A few months later, in November 1989, the two Belgian researchers appeared in a hearing room in Washington, testifying before the Special Senate Committee on Aging, which Pryor heads. Flanked by charts comparing U.S. and European prices, Adriaenssens gave the chief conclusions of the second study. "The average prices in the United States," Adriaenssens testified, "are 54 percent more expensive than the average prices in the European Economic Community." The charts showed that Americans on average were paying significantly more for drugs than even European countries with high prices.

Congress had known for years that Americans paid more than Europeans. But this was one of the few studies by an independent group that showed precisely how much more. For some drugs, the study showed, Americans were paying two or three times as much as Europeans. The price of Valium in Greece, for example, was one-tenth the U.S. price, Adriaenssens testified.

"Excuse me," Senator Pryor said. "Do you mean a U.S. citizen pays ten times the price for Valium that you pay in Greece?"

"Indeed," Adriaenssens said. "The average U.S. price is ten times the price a consumer would pay in Greece. The highest U.S. prices are fifteen times the prices in Greece."

Senator Pryor had another question. "Are American drugs, manufactured in America by American manufacturers, being sold today in these European countries at a lower price than the American consumer is buying that drug?"

"Yes, in most cases, I think," Adriaenssens said. "Over 50 percent cheaper than in the United States."

Senator Pryor asked Adriaenssens if he thought the United States should negotiate cheaper prices the way European governments do.

"Yes," Adriaenssens said. "It seems unfair to have a system in which only the producer can fix prices, and the patient or purchaser cannot negotiate."

France. Philippe Alain Joyon's pharmacy on the Rue Ernest Renan in Paris is a very authoritative and prosperous-looking store, just as Philippe Alain Joyon is a very authoritative and prosperous-looking man, dressed in a long white coat and wearing brass-rimmed glasses.

In France, where drugstores are allowed to sell only health-related products, the average pharmacist makes more than the average physician (440,000 francs a year versus 360,000). And no wonder, considering the important role drugs play in the type of medicine practiced in France.

Few doctors use as many drugs as does the French physician, who thinks nothing of prescribing five or six drugs at a time for someone coming in with a complaint as vague as dizziness or headaches. When patients get these prescriptions, they go to shops like Joyon's to have them filled, mostly at government expense, depending on the type of medicine.

The government pays the entire cost of some drugs, Joyon said, bringing out boxes of pills with white labels stamped with an "X." This label, which patients rip off and stick onto government forms they send in for reimbursement, signifies that the government will pick up the entire bill. Some packages have white labels without Xs. This means the government will pay 70 percent of the cost; others have blue labels, entitling patients to 40 percent reimbursement.

Through this reimbursement system, the government determines and imposes medical priorities for French society, which is free to disagree—at its own expense. So-called comfort drugs, for the relief of such things as pain from arthritis and varicose veins, bear blue labels. Cancer drugs are entitled to full payment; the government pays 70 percent of the cost of most heart drugs and blood pressure pills. Why more support for cancer than heart drugs?

"There are a lot more people with heart problems than cancer," Joyon said.

But why does that justify less government support?

"I don't know why," he said with a shrug. "It is a fact."

Joyon described other peculiarities of the French system. Drugs are not dispensed individually, as they are in the United States, but come from the manufacturer prepackaged, usually twenty-eight pills to the box. This is a problem, Joyon said, when physicians are just trying out a drug to see if it will work for a patient because the entire box of twenty-eight must be purchased. And it's also a problem when a physician prescribes one pill a day for a month because most months have thirty or thirty-one days. So instead of buying thirty pills, the patient must buy fifty-six.

■

A few miles from Joyon's shop, in the Hospital St. Louis, six college students are gathered around two makeshift plywood tables, sorting out boxes of partially used prescription drugs. Lined with shelves loaded with all sorts of drugs, the room looks like a hospital pharmacy except the packages have been opened.

The students are volunteers for *Pharmaciens sans frontiers*—Pharmacists Without Borders, an association of pharmacists formed to help economically poor nations. One of the group's major activities is collecting wasted drugs in France and redistributing them. The French are encouraged to bring in unused drugs to any of France's 22,000 pharmacies, which send them on to ninety collection centers around the country.

Many donated drugs are heart medicines that patients had used only a few days before being switched to other medicines, as their doctors tried to find just the right drug. The French waste so many drugs that Pharmacists Without Borders is only one of several groups collecting medicine for global redistribution.

■

Drug companies are particularly aggressive in promoting their drugs in France to make up for controlled prices. And French doctors are very willing to prescribe them, to prevent their patients, who expect a lot of drugs, from switching doctors. Government officials say France has 110,000 physicians, 30,000 more than needed, and the competition for patients is strong.

Responding to patient demands and heavily funded promotional campaigns, French doctors prescribe far more drugs than their counterparts in other European nations. Most of the French prescriptions are for higher-priced brand-name products, rather than generics. Only 2 percent to 3 percent of French prescriptions are written for generic drugs, compared with about 35 percent in the United States.

French patients expect to get prescriptions, said Paris pediatrician Remy Assathiany, who agrees that brand names are preferred in France. "Prescribing brand-name drugs is a habit," Assathiany said of himself and other doctors. "I don't know about the generics."

To avoid waste and reduce costs, the government recently launched a campaign to persuade doctors and patients to use fewer drugs. When prescribing for a month, doctors are being asked to write prescriptions for four weeks—twenty-eight days—to correspond with the number of pills in a box and avoid wasting the extra box of drugs.

Even with the overuse of medicine, just about everyone agrees—doctors, government officials, drug company representatives—that France is an austere market for the pharmaceutical industry. The drug industry says that since price controls were imposed, research and development in the French pharmaceutical industry are not as productive as they once were. No price increases have been granted by the government since 1988, and before that, prices were increasing by 1 percent to 2 percent a year, a French government official said. In the United States, until very recently drug prices increased by about 10 percent a year.

The pharmaceutical industry says price controls discourage pharmaceutical research. That's why, the industry says, countries like France have developed so few world-class drugs and the United States, with no price restrictions, has developed so many. But just about all industrialized nations have some form of price control, and many of them, such as England, have developed important drugs.

Despite the limitations in France, drug companies are eager to sell there because it is a huge market, with so many people taking so many drugs. It is a market that has been flooded with me-too drugs the French are eager to buy.

Though drug prices in France are 31 percent below the European average, according to the Belgian report, the per-capita expenditure in France is twice the average. But still it is not the highest. That honor belongs to Germany, where people not only use a lot of drugs but prices are among the highest on the continent.

Germany. Germany's per-capita drug expenditures have always been the highest in Europe—more than twice the European average. Government officials hope that is changing.

In 1989, the government passed the Health Reform Act (HRA), a radical law that imposes strict limits on how much private medical insurance companies will pay for different classes of drugs. The law's central feature is a "reference" pricing system whereby the same price is paid for similar drugs. For instance, all versions of nifedipine, a comparatively new type of heart drug, have the same reference price.

Prescription medicine is grouped into three categories: (1) medicines with the same active ingredients (the brand-name drug and all generic copies), (2) medicines with similar active ingredients, and (3) medicines that achieve the same therapeutic results, even if the ingredients are different. The reference price is set by a committee of doctors and representatives of the nation's many health-insurance plans. Drug companies, which are not represented on the committee, are free to charge above this amount, but German patients have to pay the difference between the reference price and what the manufacturers charge.

Before the HRA was enacted, cautious politicians and supporters of the pharmaceutical industry warned that patients, accustomed to "free" drugs (paid for by their insurance plans), would not tolerate extra charges. So far, the predicted protests have not happened, because the industry decided not to confront the government. As soon as the committee set a reference price, pharmaceutical companies lowered prices of their brand-name drugs in that class.

"The response of the drug companies was spectacular," said Gunnar Griesewell, an economist in the German Ministry of Health. "They even sent sales representatives out on weekends to tell doctors that the prices [of their drugs] would be coming down."

Prices fell an average of 20 percent in the first category of drugs to be indexed, said Herbert Reichelt, an economist with AOK, the biggest association of health-insurance companies in Germany.

Reichelt said that so far the pricing committee has indexed drugs representing 40 percent of the market; it hopes to increase this to 80 percent. The other 20 percent won't be indexed, he said, because the drugs are unique agents or because committee members can't agree on which ones are similar. Since 1989, the annual increase in all drug costs has ranged from 1 percent to 3 percent, half of what it had been before the new regulations. Reichelt said it is difficult to say how much of this is due to index pricing.

Reichelt said the industry has made up much of what it lost to lower reference prices by increasing the cost and promoting the use of drugs that have not been indexed. "The system is working very well," Reichelt said, "but the pharmaceutical industry is very creative in finding new ways to make money."

Still, Reichelt voiced confidence that the new system will ultimately save Germans money. What is most important, he said, is that this constitutes the first time the government has used Germany's powerful insurance industry to influence drug prices.

■

German pediatrician Juergen Bausch, like all doctors in Germany, has good reason to prescribe as economically as possible: If he goes above a certain annual limit, Bausch will be penalized by his medical association, which oversees the way health-insurance funds are used in the community.

Bausch said a German general practitioner is allowed to prescribe an average of fifty-five marks ($37) worth of medicine per patient every three-month period and 211 marks ($142) if the patient is over sixty-five. Bausch, whose practice is in Bad Soden, thirty miles outside Frankfurt, said he has never been penalized for over-prescribing but many colleagues have. "This is taken very seriously," he said.

German doctors have a variety of methods to keep pharmaceutical costs down. They can prescribe generic drugs, and many do. More than 20 percent of prescriptions in Germany are for generics. They can write "re-import" on prescriptions, which means that instead of filling the prescription with a domestically distributed product, the pharmacist will use a drug brought in from a country, such as Italy, where drugs cost 15 percent to 20 percent less than in Germany. Because of price differences between the two countries, it's cheaper to buy a drug that is first shipped to Italy and then to Germany with the Italian price than to buy a drug made in Germany.

Patients don't have to shop around because all stores in Germany must charge the same price for the same drug, though they pass on the discount for re-imported drugs to the customer. When prices are changed, the new price is faxed to all 20,000 German apothecaries, which must make the required price adjustment immediately.

Bausch, the drug specialist for the local physicians' association, said the new regulations were needed because drug companies were charging so much. But he said patients are also to blame for wanting so many drugs. "The German patient believes that if you feel sick and you take a pill, you will feel better," he said. "The patient doesn't want to hear from the doctor to stop smoking, to start eating the right food. They want the pill that will make them thin and make them happy and make them strong. They think that there is a pill to take care of everything."

Britain. British drug prices are cheaper than the Germans' and higher than the French, but overall, the English spend far less per capita on drugs. The British per-capita expenditure is less than the average for all European countries.

The British government puts no limits on drug prices or drug reimbursements, but it does put a limit on the profit companies may make on sales to the National Health Service, the primary purchaser of drugs in Britain. The government negotiates with each company individually, deciding on profit targets. That allows drug companies to set prices comparable to, or even higher than, in European countries but still less than prices in the United States. Over time, differences between U.S. and British prices widen considerably because prices in Britain rarely increase once set. Jo Walton, a financial analyst in London with Lehman Bros. International, said a comparative study done by her firm in 1991 showed that U.S. prices averaged 80 percent more than those in the United Kingdom.

The British government also discourages drug companies from spending more than 9 percent of their British sales on marketing and promotion through its profit-control scheme. This is less than one-half of what firms spend on promotion in the United States. Such a restriction in the United States would cut the industry's operating costs by roughly $5 billion a year. The goal of Britain's pharmaceutical price regulation plan, said one government official, is to provide companies with enough profit to encourage R&D and investment in the United Kingdom, while protecting the public from exorbitant prices.

"In Britain there is an uneasy balance between the consumer voice and the industry voice," said Allan Maynard, a health economist at the University of York. "The industry voice is very organized and targeted, the consumer voice is poorly targeted and more diverse." Maynard said the government favors industry because it wants the jobs and the favorable balance of trade the industry provides.

The British success in keeping down per-capita drug expenditures, however, is only partly due to its regulation system. An equally important factor is the British doctor/patient attitude toward drugs. They don't use as many drugs as doctors and patients in other countries.

■

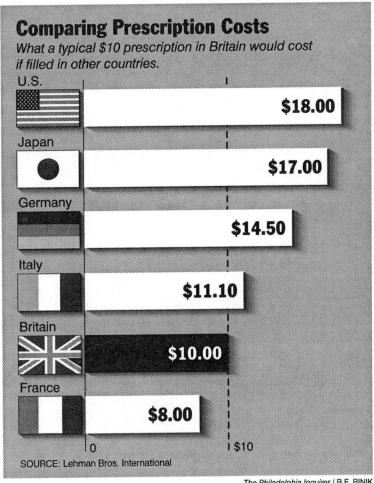

Comparing Prescription Costs
*What a typical $10 prescription in Britain would cost
if filled in other countries.*

U.S. $18.00

Japan $17.00

Germany $14.50

Italy $11.10

Britain $10.00

France $8.00

0                    $10

SOURCE: Lehman Bros. International

The Philadelphia Inquirer / B.F. BINIK

The office of London general practitioner Marc Rowland is a sparse room with an examining table, two metal chairs, a metal desk, and a computer with a printer, to produce prescriptions. The patients are called from the waiting room by an electric sign that flashes their number when Rowland is ready to see them. They enter the office, describe what's bothering them, answer a few questions, get advice and sometimes a prescription, and leave. Patients seem satisfied with this. The exchanges are cordial and there's no sense of rushing, but rarely does a visit last more than six minutes.

The therapy offered by British doctors is as economical as these office visits are brief. British doctors often counsel their patients to do nothing but wait for the problem to heal itself, or to use home remedies rather than expensive drugs (Rowland advises warm olive oil to treat ear wax) or to avoid treatments that have not been proved worthwhile (Rowland is slow to prescribe anti-cholesterol drugs). The British system is "ruthlessly driven by what's been proved," Rowland said.

British patients don't expect to have long encounters with doctors. And they don't expect to leave their doctors' offices with prescriptions for expensive drugs. Rowland believes this has more to do with culture and the British character than the penny-pinching nature of the National Health Service. "The British patient seems to be quite accepting of the idea that it is not necessary to order a lot of drugs to do good medicine," Rowland said. This is not so true on the continent, he said, especially France. Rowland said he routinely prescribes more drugs than he thinks necessary for his French patients so they won't be offended.

Judging from Rowland's practice, it would seem unnecessary, but in 1991 the National Health Service started monitoring the prescribing habits of private practitioners to "help achieve cost-effective and rational prescribing," as a government pamphlet put it. Every three months, Rowland receives a computer printout from the Prescription Pricing Authority with comparative bar charts showing how many drugs he prescribed during that period. The charts compare his prescribing with other doctors in his practice, the national average for all doctors in England, and other patients with the same kinds of conditions. The printout also shows the number and average cost of his prescriptions. Doctors who consistently prescribe above the norm for their practice or region are visited by someone from the National Health Service and in extreme cases can be fined, although so far this hasn't happened.

It is not clear whether it's because of the NHS surveillance or the pricing scheme or the British medical training or the English character, but something seems to be working in Britain. Not only does the country spend little on drugs, it is considered one of the best environments in the world for pharmaceutical R&D, having contributed many of the most important drugs ever developed.

Pharmaceutical executives in the United States say the studies showing that drugs often cost substantially more here than abroad are misleading if they suggest the drug industry is taking advantage of American consumers. The executives say price differences are explained by a variety of factors, such as differences in the currency exchange rate, Europe's faster and cheaper drug-approval systems, and the less litigious nature of Europeans.

"We always set out to price our products at similar levels from country to country," Merck chief executive officer P. Roy Vagelos said in a *Science* journal article, which company representatives cited when asked for Merck comment. "But variations in government price controls, exchange rates, dates of new drug approval, health care financing practices, and other factors tend to result in different prices for different countries."

Said Fred Telling, vice president for planning and policy for U.S. Pharmaceuticals Group of Pfizer Inc.: "The U.S. provides the best opportunity for pharmaceutical firms to appropriately price products, recognizing the relatively short product life that compounds have before they become available generically. . . . Product prices are heavily related to policies and markets in which those prices emerge. Many other countries have various forms of price regulations."

Citing figures from the Organization for Economic Cooperation and Development (OECD), a twenty-four-nation intergovernmental agency, the Pharmaceutical Manufacturers Association said that "U.S. per-capita expenditures on pharmaceuticals are about average for an industrialized country. . . ." The OECD charts showed that Americans spent an average of $210 for drugs in 1990, which was less than the $220 spent in Italy, $230 spent in France, and $257 spent in Germany.

Moreover, the Pharmaceutical Manufacturers Association said, the average American worked fewer hours to earn the money to buy drugs than workers in other nations. Citing OECD and U.S. Labor Department statistics, the industry trade association said the typical U.S. wage-earner worked 14.2 hours in 1991 to earn the money to pay for a year's supply of drugs. This compared with 17.3 hours for Italians, 19.8 hours for Germans, and 20.4 hours for the French.

The implication of these statistics is that Americans are way ahead of Europeans when it comes to buying drugs. But Jean-Pierre Poullier of Paris does not agree. Poullier is the OECD medical economist who helped provide many of the figures on which the Pharmaceutical Manufacturers Association's comments are based.

Poullier said that not only are American drug prices among the highest of the twenty-four OECD nations, they have been rising faster than any other nation's. He said exchange rates, government regulations, the cost of lawsuits, and other factors cited play a relatively small role in the high U.S. prices. Drugs are cheaper in Europe because they're controlled in Europe.

He said the reason Americans' annual drug bills are slightly less than those of the French, Italians, or Germans is that, on a *per capita basis,*

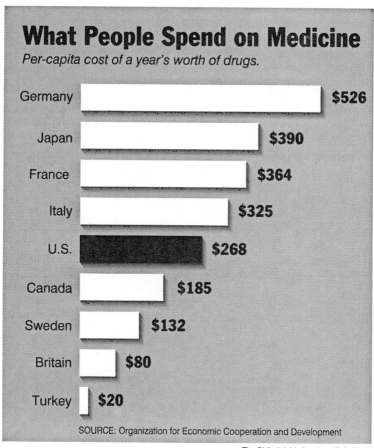

What People Spend on Medicine
Per-capita cost of a year's worth of drugs.

Germany	$526
Japan	$390
France	$364
Italy	$325
U.S.	$268
Canada	$185
Sweden	$132
Britain	$80
Turkey	$20

SOURCE: Organization for Economic Cooperation and Development

The Philadelphia Inquirer / B.F. BINIK

Americans buy one-half to one-third as many drugs. At 250 million, the United States has a population many times larger than Italy, France, or Germany, and Americans' drugs are not covered by a national health plan. He speculated that Europeans would probably use fewer drugs, too, if they had to pay U.S. prices. Poullier said this also explains in part why Americans work fewer hours to pay for prescription medicine. They buy fewer drugs. Also, U.S. salaries are higher and have significantly more buying power than those in Europe.

Poullier said fifteen studies have been done comparing international drug prices, and they all show the same thing: U.S. prices are highest.

Dressed in conservative business suits with fake identification badges pinned to their jackets and with chains and handcuffs in their pockets, a handful of AIDS activists strode onto the balcony overlooking the floor of the New York Stock Exchange. The plan was to disrupt the exchange and gain worldwide media attention for their protests against the Burroughs Wellcome Co. The drug company was charging $8,000 a year for AZT (Retrovir), which at the time, in 1989, was the only drug proved effective against the AIDS virus.

Just before the bell sounded to signal the start of another day on the trading floor, the activists whipped out chains and handcuffed themselves to a banister while compatriots blared away with air horns. Startled security guards rushed to arrest the intruders while still other activists took photographs, which were rushed to the Associated Press. Within less than an hour, the photographs were transmitted to newspapers and broadcast stations throughout the world.

Masters at drawing attention from the media, the activists from Act Up, an AIDS protest group, had conducted another foray in their ongoing fight against the high prices of AIDS drugs. Not long afterward, Burroughs Wellcome reduced the price of AZT.

Drug companies have come under increasing pressure in the United States to hold down prices, and they have begun to respond. Seven major companies have announced they will hold price increases within the rate of inflation.

In doing so, they were taking the advice of P. Roy Vagelos, the chairman and chief executive officer of Merck & Co., who warned in 1991 that if drug companies didn't restrain prices, the government might. "It is clear that the U.S. public and our congressmen and senators are focusing on health care costs," Vagelos told a gathering of securities analysts in November 1991. "I detest regulation, but it may be brought on" by rising drug prices, he said.

Most of the public pressure has been aimed at helping specific segments of the population, such as AIDS patients. Unlike European governments, the U.S. government has done little to protect the general population from high drug prices.

The Europeans began to control prices after World War II, when a social consensus for government-financed national health care grew in England and Europe. Once this happened, the government became involved with the economics of health care in a "big way," said David Taylor, a fellow in health policy analysis at the Kings Fund Institute,

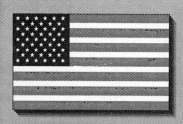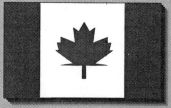

Comparing Prices: U.S. and Canada

*All prices are for bottles of 100 pills
except where otherwise stated.*

U.S. manufacturer	Condition	Price U.S.[1]	Price Canada[2]	% difference
Amoxil (SmithKline Beecham)	infections	$17.27	$16.46	5%
Lanoxin (Burroughs Wellcome)	cardiovascular system	$7.83	$6.75	16%
Zantac* (Glaxo)	ulcers	$70.19	$53.82	30%
Premarin (Wyeth Ayerst)	osteoporosis	$26.47	$10.10	162%
Xanax (Upjohn)	anxiety	$47.81	$16.92	183%
Cardizem (Marion)	cardiovascular system	$49.00	$57.51	−15%
Synthroid (Boots)	thyroid	$11.80	$3.13	278%
Ceclor (Eli Lilly & Co.)	infections	$134.18	$84.14	59%
Vasotec (Merck & Co.)	cardiovascular system	$66.90	$78.75	−15%
Tenormin(ICI)	cardiovascular system	$61.68	$47.34	30%
Procardia (Pfizer Inc.)	cardiovascular system	$39.46	$42.14	−6%
Ortho-novum** (Ortho)	birth control	$16.00	$8.75	83%
Capoten (Bristol-Meyers Squibb)	cardiovascular system	$41.73	$43.36	−4%
Naprosyn (Syntex)	arthritis	$72.36	$42.64	70%
Tagamet (SmithKline Beecham)	ulcers	$57.16	$34.27	67%

*60 pills
**28 pills

[1] Wholesale, May 1991
[2] Feb. 1991

SOURCE: General Accounting Office

The Philadelphia Inquirer / B.F. BINIK

a London-based think tank. With worldwide medical inflation, it was only a matter of time before budget-conscious governments looked for ways to control medical costs, including drug prices, he said

At first, the British National Health Service did nothing to limit drug prices, he said, but as economic conditions tightened, so did government-instituted controls. This has happened throughout Europe, most recently in Germany when the government, concerned about increases in the cost of government-regulated health insurance, established the price-indexing system.

"If you don't have a national health system, there's no necessity for the government to control prices," said L.G. Thomas 3d, associate professor of organization and management at Emory University Business School. As Thomas sees it, it's more a matter of "procurement" than regulation, meaning that when the government is the purchaser, it has a vested interest in keeping prices down.

Other experts think that the reason the United States and European countries reacted differently in their approach stems from far more basic issues rooted in the culture and political expectations of the people. Americans are much more wary of the government setting prices for anything and think that any attempts to do this smacks of socialism or communism, said Guy Sermeus, the Belgian economist who compared U.S. and European drug prices. "Such things as pricing controls are more tolerated in Europe," Sermeus said, adding that Europeans don't "automatically correlate controls with the socialistic system."

Uwe E. Reinhardt, a Princeton University professor of economics specializing in medical matters, said that in the United States, drugs are viewed as "private consumption goods, like hair spray," whereas in Europe they're considered necessities that should be financed by insurance or the government. Even with necessities, Americans don't want the government to step in unless the cost of that necessity becomes a major part of their budget, he said. Reinhardt believes this may be happening with drugs. As far back as 1981, he had addressed meetings of drug company executives, warning that they were "driving their industry into the socialized corner" with continued price increases.

Reinhardt said he did not think it likely that the U.S. government would attempt to control drug prices, at least not yet. A national health system, or the growing purchasing power of health maintenance organizations, might be enough to slow drug price inflation. But if they don't, controls might be considered.

The most far-reaching attempt by the government to do something has come from Sen. David Pryor (D., Ark.), who in 1990 pushed through the first federal law requiring companies to discount drugs sold under the government-funded Medicaid program.

Large buying groups also are starting to fight back. Hospital chains, HMOs, and insurance companies have forced price concessions by setting up formularies, listing specific drugs that staff doctors may prescribe. To get their medicines on the formularies, drug companies must compete, by offering low prices.

Major corporations, with huge labor forces and expensive health plans, are turning to firms that specialize in managing employee prescription-benefit programs as a way to reduce drug costs. Others are requiring employees with chronic medical conditions to buy their drugs from large mail-order companies, which usually offer cheaper prices. Drug utilization review is also becoming increasingly popular as a way for companies to hold down costs. These are systems to promote the cost-effective and proper use of drugs through watchdog companies that monitor how doctors write prescriptions.

In Pennsylvania, for example, each month the state PACE program, which subsidizes prescription drugs for older persons from state lottery earnings, reviews the amount and kinds of drugs taken by its members. PACE staff members notify doctors when they see instances of overmedication or use of multiple drugs where adverse interactions are likely. The PACE program has refused to reimburse pharmacies for medication if a drug appears to be inappropriate for the patient.

Some organizations are trying to counteract drug company promotion with "counter-sales representatives." In Massachusetts, Blue Cross and Blue Shield is sending representatives to doctors' offices to provide impartial information about the drugs they prescribe. In California, teams of pharmacists from Kaiser Permanente, a large health care system, visit with physicians to update them on the latest in cost-effective prescribing. In Michigan, a hospital banned drug company salespeople in protest of high prices.

At best, though, the various cost-containment strategies are merely shifting costs from one segment of society to another. European countries hold down drug costs, and as a result the international companies seek their biggest profits in the United States, where there are no controls. HMOs and hospitals force price concessions from the manufacturers, and the prices in retail drugstores continue to climb. Federal legislation opens the market to generic companies, and brand-name companies raise prices to make up for lost sales. Medicaid patients get a break, and everyone else pays higher prices.

If the drug companies can't make it in one place, they will make it in another.

Epilogue

A consensus is growing that something must be done to contain health care costs, including drug prices. But there is little consensus on how to do it. There is particularly strong disagreement between those inside and outside the industry.

The outsiders suggest that the dynamics of the marketplace be changed to give consumers a better chance to use buying power as a leverage on prices, the way it works with most consumer purchases.

Harvard Medical School professor Jerry Avorn said the most "doable" way of controlling rising drug costs would be to provide physicians with better information on the best and most cost-effective drugs. "It's got to be someone's responsibility to make this information available," he said. "If we as a society leave it up to the manufacturers of drugs to be the only purveyors of information about drugs, then we shouldn't expect them to do anything but to try to increase sales."

Senator David Pryor (D., Ark.) has proposed a National Pharmacy and Therapeutics Committee, composed of physicians and scientists, who would determine which drugs were therapeutically equivalent. Doctors then could choose the cheapest drugs with the confidence that they would be as effective as more expensive ones. Buyers then could use this information to try to negotiate a better deal. And health-insurance plans could peg their payments to the prices of the listed drugs, similar to what the Germans are doing with their price indexing. Currently, most comparative studies on drugs are funded by the industry, which has an obvious self-interest.

Looking at it from the patient's point of view, Abbey Meyers, executive director of the National Organization for Rare Disorders, called for federal controls. "The government keeps talking about a free market and a level playing field," she said. "It's the government that hasn't recognized that we are in a world economy. And the United States should maintain control over health care costs, as every other country does."

Tom Snedden, director of the PACE program in Pennsylvania, thinks the consumer must be given a financial reason to seek cheaper drug prices. "Where the industry has been so successful," he said, "is in seeing that the consumer doesn't have a vested interest. The costs are out of control because third parties are paying for health care." He said patients need to be better educated about what drugs can and cannot do so they will stop demanding medicine they don't need, such as antibiotics, which are useless against the common cold.

David Banks, who spent four years reviewing drug advertising for the Food and Drug Administration, thinks the public needs to be told how the drug industry manipulates information to suit its commercial interests. "The problem is that drug companies have gotten too good at disguising their biased and misleading promotional activities," he said. "The likely result may be medical care that is unnecessary, inferior, needlessly expensive, and counter to the best interests of all except the drug companies."

Some government leaders have suggested a board or commission to oversee prices, in much the same way that public utility rates are regulated. Others say the Food and Drug Administration could be given the power to deny approval to new drugs that offer neither a therapeutic nor economic advantage over existing drugs, as the Norwegians do.

Those within the industry bridle at such suggestions and warn of dire consequences from such meddling.

"I don't think there is any question that it would cut back the amount being invested in research and development," said Gerald J. Mossinghoff, president of the Pharmaceutical Manufacturers Association. "You would have less new drugs coming out. You would have less breakthroughs."

"Remember, our entire society is set up in order to drive economic return," said Kurt Landgraff, executive vice president of Du Pont Merck Pharmaceutical Co. "If you want a pharmaceutical industry that is making decisions based on other-than-economic realities, that is where you need constructive dialogue between the government, the pharmaceutical industry, academic and regulatory environment—we need to talk in the same room."

And Robert C. Black, president of the U.S. pharmaceutical unit of ICI of Great Britain, said, "If you want to start playing a price-spiral game, which is cutting price and someone else cuts price, pretty soon you will be in the commodity generic marketplace, and we will go bankrupt pretty quickly. If you play that game, you will not be able to support all that research effort. Instead of talking about the pharmaceutical industry as the most profitable industry in the country, we ought to turn it around and figure out what happened to the rest of American industry, that it is so unprofitable. One thing about having an industry that is profitable: We have been able to invest in R&D. We have been able to maintain a positive balance of trade. And we are competitive globally. There are not too many industries in this country that can say that."

The message from industry is very consistent, very loud, and very clear: The drugs of tomorrow are dependent on keeping this the most profitable business in America.

And the message from the consumer?

"I look at it as taxation without representation," said Norrie Thomas, who runs a benefits program in Minneapolis. "They can charge anything they want for a drug because they spend so much for R&D. We don't have any say."

Appendix 1

How to write or telephone your lawmakers

Following is a list of senators and representatives in the 103rd Congress, as well as the names and addresses of key committees that deal with health-care issues, including prescription drugs. The information in this list comes from *Congressional Quarterly* and was current as of January 14, 1993.

■

House and Senate members have offices in six buildings in Washington; those buildings are designated in the listings below by their initials. Here are the full names of the buildings that the initials refer to, followed by the appropriate addresses.

SHOB:
Senate Hart Office Building
Washington, DC 20510

CHOB:
Cannon House Office Building
Washington, DC 20515

LHOB:
Longworth House Office Building
Washington, DC 20515

SROB:
Senate Russell Office Building
Washington, DC 20510

RHOB:
Rayburn House Office Building
Washington, DC 20515

DOB:
Dirksen Office Building
Washington, DC 20515

In the following committee listings, all phone numbers are in area code 202.

Committees dealing with health-care issues

	Room	Bldg.	Tele.
U.S. SENATE			
Special Committee on Aging			
Chairman: Sen. David H. Pryor (D., Ark.)	G-31	DOB	224-5364
Committee on Labor and Human Resources			
Chairman: Sen. Edward M. Kennedy (D., Mass.)	428	DOB	224-5375
Senate Committee on Finance, Subcommittee on Health for Families and the Uninsured			
Chairman: Sen. Donald W. Riegle (D., Mich.)	205	DOB	224-4515

	Room	Bldg.	Tele.
HOUSE OF REPRESENTATIVES			
House Select Committee on Aging			
Chairman: William J. Hughes (D., N.J.)	712 Annex 1		226-3375
Committee on Energy and Commerce, Subcommittee on Health and the Environment			
Chairman: Rep. Henry A. Waxman (D., Calif.)	2424	RHOB	225-0130
Committee on Energy and Commerce			
Chairman: Rep. John D. Dingell (D., Mich.)	2125	RHOB	225-2927
House Ways and Means Committee, Subcommittee on Health			
Chairman: Rep. Pete Stark (D., Calif.)	1114	LHOB	225-7785
Committee on Appropriations, Subcommittee on Agriculture, Rural Development, Food and Drug Administration, and Related Agencies			
Chairman: Rep. Richard Durbin (D., Ill.)	2362	RHOB	225-2638

Following, by state, is a listing of all senators and representatives in the 103rd Congress. Each line has the official's name, party designation, district number (for representatives only), office number and building, and telephone number. All telephone numbers are in area code 202. The designation AL signifies that the representative serves an at-large district.

Name Party	Dist.	Room	Bldg.	Tele.
ALABAMA				
Senators				
Howell Heflin (D)		728	SHOB	224-4124
Richard C. Shelby (D)		313	SHOB	224-5744
Representatives				
Sonny Callahan (R)	1st	2418	RHOB	225-4931
Terry Everett (R)	2nd	208	CHOB	225-2901
Glen Browder (D)	3rd	1221	LHOB	225-3261
Tom Bevill (D)	4th	2302	RHOB	225-4876
Bud Cramer (D)	5th	1318	LHOB	225-4801
Spencer Bachus (R)	6th	216	CHOB	225-4921
Earl F. Hilliard (D)	7th	1007	LHOB	225-2665
ALASKA				
Senators				
Ted Stevens (R)		522	SHOB	224-3004
Frank H. Murkowski (R)		709	SHOB	224-6665
Representative				
Don Young (R)	AL	2331	RHOB	225-5765
AMERICAN SAMOA				
Representative				
Eni F.H. Faleomavaega (D)	AL	109	CHOB	225-8577
ARIZONA				
Senators				
Dennis DeConcini (D)		328	SHOB	224-4521
John McCain (R)		111	SROB	224-2235
Representatives				
Sam Coppersmith (D)	1st	1607	LHOB	225-2635
Ed Pastor (D)	2nd	408	CHOB	225-4065
Bob Stump (R)	3rd	211	CHOB	225-4576
Jon Kyl (R)	4th	2440	RHOB	225-3361
Jim Kolbe (R)	5th	405	CHOB	225-2542
Karan English (D)	6th	1223	LHOB	225-2190
ARKANSAS				
Senators				
Dale Bumpers (D)		229	DOB	224-4843
David Pryor (D)		267	SROB	224-2353
Representatives				
Blanche Lambert (D)	1st	1204	LHOB	225-4076
Ray Thornton (D)	2nd	1214	LHOB	225-2506
Tim Hutchinson (R)	3rd	1541	LHOB	225-4301
Jay Dickey (R)	4th	1338	LHOB	225-3772
CALIFORNIA				
Senators				
Dianne Feinstein (D)		367	DOB	224-3841
Barbara Boxer (D)		112	SHOB	224-3553
Representatives				
Dan Hamburg (D)	1st	114	CHOB	225-3311
Wally Herger (R)	2nd	2433	RHOB	225-3076
Vic Fazio (D)	3rd	2113	RHOB	225-5716
John T. Doolittle (R)	4th	1524	LHOB	225-2511

Name Party	Dist.	Room	Bldg.	Tele.
Robert T. Matsui (D)	5th	2311	RHOB	225-7163
Lynn Woolsey (D)	6th	439	CHOB	225-5161
George Miller (D)	7th	2205	RHOB	225-2095
Nancy Pelosi (D)	8th	240	CHOB	225-4965
Ronald V. Dellums (D)	9th	2136	RHOB	225-2661
Bill Baker (R)	10th	1724	LHOB	225-1880
Richard W. Pombo (R)	11th	1519	LHOB	225-1947
Tom Lantos (D)	12th	2182	RHOB	225-3531
Pete Stark (D)	13th	239	CHOB	225-5065
Anna G. Eshoo (D)	14th	1505	LHOB	225-8104
Norman Y. Mineta (D)	15th	2221	RHOB	225-2631
Don Edwards (D)	16th	2307	RHOB	225-3072
Leon E. Panetta (D)	17th	339	CHOB	225-2861
Gary Condit (D)	18th	1123	LHOB	225-6131
Richard H. Lehman (D)	19th	1226	LHOB	225-4540
Calvin Dooley (D)	20th	1227	LHOB	225-3341
Bill Thomas (R)	21st	2209	RHOB	225-2915
Michael Huffington (R)	22nd	113	CHOB	225-3601
Elton Gallegly (R)	23rd	2441	RHOB	225-5811
Anthony C. Beilenson (D)	24th	2465	RHOB	225-5911
Howard P. "Buck" McKeon (R)	25th	307	CHOB	225-1956
Howard L. Berman (D)	26th	2201	RHOB	225-4695
Carlos J. Moorhead (R)	27th	2346	RHOB	225-4176
David Dreier (R)	28th	411	CHOB	225-2305
Henry A. Waxman (D)	29th	2408	RHOB	225-3976
Xavier Becerra (D)	30th	1710	LHOB	225-6235
Matthew G. Martinez (D)	31st	2231	RHOB	225-5464
Julian C. Dixon (D)	32nd	2400	RHOB	225-7084
Lucille Roybal-Allard (D)	33rd	1717	LHOB	225-1766
Esteban E. Torres (D)	34th	1740	LHOB	225-5256
Maxine Waters (D)	35th	1207	LHOB	225-2201
Jane Harman (D)	36th	325	CHOB	225-8220
Walter R. Tucker (D)	37th	419	CHOB	225-7924
Steve Horn (R)	38th	1023	LHOB	225-6676
Ed Royce (R)	39th	1404	LHOB	225-4111
Jerry Lewis (R)	40th	2312	RHOB	225-5861
Jay C. Kim (R)	41st	502	CHOB	225-3201
George E. Brown, Jr. (D)	42nd	2300	RHOB	225-6161
Ken Calvert (R)	43rd	1523	LHOB	225-1986
Al McCandless (R)	44th	2422	RHOB	225-5330
Dana Rohrabacher (R)	45th	1027	LHOB	225-2415
Robert K. Dornan (R)	46th	2402	RHOB	225-2965
C. Christopher Cox (R)	47th	206	CHOB	225-5611
Ron Packard (R)	48th	2162	RHOB	225-3906
Lynn Schenk (D)	49th	315	CHOB	225-2040
Bob Filner (D)	50th	504	CHOB	225-8045
Randy "Duke" Cunningham (R)	51st	117	CHOB	225-5452
Duncan Hunter (R)	52nd	133	CHOB	225-5672
COLORADO				
Senators				
Hank Brown (R)		717	SHOB	224-5941
Ben Nighthorse Campbell (D)		380	SROB	224-5852

Name Party	Dist.	Room	Bldg.	Tele.
Representatives				
Patricia Schroeder (D)	1st	2208	RHOB	225-4431
David E. Skaggs (D)	2nd	1124	LHOB	225-2161
Scott McInnis (R)	3rd	512	CHOB	225-4761
Wayne Allard (R)	4th	422	CHOB	225-4676
Joel Hefley (R)	5th	2442	RHOB	225-4422
Dan Schaefer (R)	6th	2448	RHOB	225-7882
CONNECTICUT				
Senators				
Christopher J. Dodd (D)		444	SROB	224-2823
Joseph I. Lieberman (D)		502	SHOB	224-4041
Representatives				
Barbara B. Kennelly (D)	1st	201	CHOB	225-2265
Sam Gejdenson (D)	2nd	2416	RHOB	225-2076
Rosa DeLauro (D)	3rd	327	CHOB	225-3661
Christopher Shays (R)	4th	1034	LHOB	225-5541
Gary Franks (R)	5th	435	CHOB	225-3822
Nancy L. Johnson (R)	6th	343	CHOB	225-4476
DELAWARE				
Senators				
William V. Roth, Jr. (R)		104	SHOB	224-2441
Joseph R. Biden, Jr. (D)		221	SROB	224-5042
Representative				
Michael N. Castle (R)	AL	1205	LHOB	225-4165
DISTRICT OF COLUMBIA				
Representative				
Eleanor Holmes Norton (D)	AL	1415	LHOB	225-8050
FLORIDA				
Senators				
Bob Graham (D)		241	DOB	224-3041
Connie Mack (R)		517	SHOB	224-5274
Representatives				
Earl Hutto (D)	1st	2435	RHOB	225-4136
Pete Peterson (D)	2nd	426	CHOB	225-5235
Corrine Brown (D)	3rd	1037	LHOB	225-0123
Tillie Fowler (R)	4th	413	CHOB	225-2501
Karen L. Thurman (D)	5th	130	CHOB	225-1002
Cliff Stearns (R)	6th	332	CHOB	225-5744
John L. Mica (R)	7th	427	CHOB	225-4035
Bill McCollum (R)	8th	2266	RHOB	225-2176
Michael Bilirakis (R)	9th	2240	RHOB	225-5755
C.W. Bill Young (R)	10th	2407	RHOB	225-5961
Sam M. Gibbons (D)	11th	2204	RHOB	225-3376
Charles T. Canady (R)	12th	1107	LHOB	225-1252
Dan Miller (R)	13th	510	CHOB	225-5015
Porter J. Goss (R)	14th	330	CHOB	225-2536
Jim Bacchus (D)	15th	432	CHOB	225-3671
Tom Lewis (R)	16th	2351	RHOB	225-5792
Carrie Meek (D)	17th	404	CHOB	225-4506
Ileana Ros-Lehtinen (R)	18th	127	CHOB	225-3931
Harry A. Johnston (D)	19th	204	CHOB	225-3001
Peter Deutsch (D)	20th	425	CHOB	225-7931
Lincoln Diaz-Balart (R)	21st	509	CHOB	225-4211
E. Clay Shaw, Jr. (R)	22nd	2267	RHOB	225-3026
Alcee L. Hastings (D)	23rd	1039	LHOB	225-1313
GEORGIA				
Senators				
Sam Nunn (D)		303	DOB	224-3521
Paul Coverdell (R)		204	SROB	224-3643
Representatives				
Jack Kingston (R)	1st	1229	LHOB	225-5831
Sanford Bishop (D)	2nd	1632	LHOB	225-3631
Mac Collins (R)	3rd	1118	LHOB	225-5901
John Linder (R)	4th	1605	LHOB	225-4272
John Lewis (D)	5th	329	CHOB	225-3801
Newt Gingrich (R)	6th	2428	RHOB	225-4501
George "Buddy" Darden (D)	7th	2303	RHOB	225-2931
J. Roy Rowland (D)	8th	2134	RHOB	225-6531
Nathan Deal (D)	9th	1406	LHOB	225-5211
Don Johnson (D)	10th	226	CHOB	225-4101
Cynthia McKinney (D)	11th	124	CHOB	225-1605
GUAM				
Representative				
Robert Anacletus Underwood (D)	AL	507	CHOB	225-1188
HAWAII				
Senators				
Daniel K. Inouye (D)		722	SHOB	224-3934
Daniel K. Akaka (D)		720	SHOB	224-6361
Representatives				
Neil Abercrombie (D)	1st	1440	LHOB	225-2726
Patsy T. Mink (D)	2nd	2135	RHOB	225-4906
IDAHO				
Senators				
Larry E. Craig (R)		302	SHOB	224-2752
Dirk Kempthorne (R)		B40	DOB	224-6142
Representatives				
Larry LaRocco (D)	1st	1117	LHOB	225-6611
Michael D. Crapo (R)	2nd	437	CHOB	225-5531
ILLINOIS				
Senators				
Paul Simon (D)		462	DOB	224-2152
Carol Moseley-Braun (D)		708	SHOB	224-2854
Representatives				
Bobby L. Rush (D)	1st	1725	LHOB	225-4372
Mel Reynolds (D)	2nd	514	CHOB	225-0773
William O. Lipinski (D)	3rd	1501	LHOB	225-5701
Luis V. Gutierrez (D)	4th	1208	LHOB	225-8203
Dan Rostenkowski (D)	5th	2111	RHOB	225-4061
Henry J. Hyde (R)	6th	2110	RHOB	225-4561
Cardiss Collins (D)	7th	2308	RHOB	225-5006
Philip M. Crane (R)	8th	233	CHOB	225-3711

Name Party	Dist.	Room	Bldg.	Tele.
Sidney R. Yates (D)	9th	2109	RHOB	225-2111
John Porter (R)	10th	1026	LHOB	225-4835
George E. Sangmeister (D)	11th	1032	LHOB	225-3635
Jerry F. Costello (D)	12th	119	CHOB	225-5661
Harris W. Fawell (R)	13th	2342	RHOB	225-3515
Dennis Hastert (R)	14th	2453	RHOB	225-2976
Thomas W. Ewing (R)	15th	1317	LHOB	225-2371
Donald Manzullo (R)	16th	506	CHOB	225-5676
Lane Evans (D)	17th	2335	RHOB	225-5905
Robert H. Michel (R)	18th	2112	RHOB	225-6201
Glenn Poshard (D)	19th	107	CHOB	225-5201
Richard J. Durbin (D)	20th	129	CHOB	225-5271

INDIANA
Senators
Name Party	Dist.	Room	Bldg.	Tele.
Richard G. Lugar (R)		306	SHOB	224-4814
Daniel R. Coats (R)		404	SROB	224-5623

Representatives
Name Party	Dist.	Room	Bldg.	Tele.
Peter J. Visclosky (D)	1st	2464	RHOB	225-2461
Philip R. Sharp (D)	2nd	2217	RHOB	225-3021
Tim Roemer (D)	3rd	415	CHOB	225-3915
Jill L. Long (D)	4th	1513	LHOB	225-4436
Steve Buyer (R)	5th	1419	LHOB	225-5037
Dan Burton (R)	6th	2411	RHOB	225-2276
John T. Myers (R)	7th	2372	RHOB	225-5805
Frank McCloskey (D)	8th	306	CHOB	225-4636
Lee H. Hamilton (D)	9th	2187	RHOB	225-5315
Andrew Jacobs, Jr. (D)	10th	2313	RHOB	225-4011

IOWA
Senators
Name Party	Dist.	Room	Bldg.	Tele.
Charles E. Grassley (R)		135	SHOB	224-3744
Tom Harkin (D)		531	SHOB	224-3254

Representatives
Name Party	Dist.	Room	Bldg.	Tele.
Jim Leach (R)	1st	2186	RHOB	225-6576
Jim Nussle (R)	2nd	308	CHOB	225-2911
Jim Ross Lightfoot (R)	3rd	2444	RHOB	225-3806
Neal Smith (D)	4th	2373	RHOB	225-4426
Fred Grandy (R)	5th	418	CHOB	225-5476

KANSAS
Senators
Name Party	Dist.	Room	Bldg.	Tele.
Bob Dole (R)		141	SHOB	224-6521
Nancy Landon Kassebaum (R)		302	SROB	224-4774

Representatives
Name Party	Dist.	Room	Bldg.	Tele.
Pat Roberts (R)	1st	1125	LHOB	225-2715
Jim Slattery (D)	2nd	2243	RHOB	225-6601
Jan Meyers (R)	3rd	2338	RHOB	225-2865
Dan Glickman (D)	4th	2371	RHOB	225-6216

KENTUCKY
Senators
Name Party	Dist.	Room	Bldg.	Tele.
Wendell H. Ford (D)		173A	SROB	224-4343
Mitch McConnell (R)		120	SROB	224-2541

Representatives
Name Party	Dist.	Room	Bldg.	Tele.
Tom Barlow (D)	1st	1408	LHOB	225-3115
William H. Natcher (D)	2nd	2333	RHOB	225-3501
Romano L. Mazzoli (D)	3rd	2246	RHOB	225-5401
Jim Bunning (R)	4th	2437	RHOB	225-3465
Harold Rogers (R)	5th	2468	RHOB	225-4601
Scotty Baesler (D)	6th	508	CHOB	225-4706

LOUISIANA
Senators
Name Party	Dist.	Room	Bldg.	Tele.
J. Bennett Johnston (D)		136	SHOB	224-5824
John B. Breaux (D)		516	SHOB	224-4623

Representatives
Name Party	Dist.	Room	Bldg.	Tele.
Robert L. Livingston (R)	1st	2368	RHOB	225-3015
William J. Jefferson (D)	2nd	428	CHOB	225-6636
W.J. "Billy" Tauzin (D)	3rd	2330	RHOB	225-4031
Cleo Fields (D)	4th	513	CHOB	225-8490
Jim McCrery (R)	5th	225	CHOB	225-2777
Richard H. Baker (R)	6th	434	CHOB	225-3901
Jimmy Hayes (D)	7th	2432	RHOB	225-2031

MAINE
Senators
Name Party	Dist.	Room	Bldg.	Tele.
William S. Cohen (R)		322	SHOB	224-2523
George J. Mitchell (D)		176	SROB	224-5344

Representatives
Name Party	Dist.	Room	Bldg.	Tele.
Thomas H. Andrews (D)	1st	1530	LHOB	225-6116
Olympia J. Snowe (R)	2nd	2268	RHOB	225-6306

MARYLAND
Senators
Name Party	Dist.	Room	Bldg.	Tele.
Paul S. Sarbanes (D)		309	SHOB	224-4524
Barbara A. Mikulski (D)		320	SHOB	224-4654

Representatives
Name Party	Dist.	Room	Bldg.	Tele.
Wayne T. Gilchrest (R)	1st	412	CHOB	225-5311
Helen Delich Bentley (R)	2nd	1610	LHOB	225-3061
Benjamin L. Cardin (D)	3rd	227	CHOB	225-4016
Albert R. Wynn (D)	4th	423	CHOB	225-8699
Steny H. Hoyer (D)	5th	1705	LHOB	225-4131
Roscoe G. Bartlett (R)	6th	312	CHOB	225-2721
Kweisi Mfume (D)	7th	2419	RHOB	225-4741
Constance A. Morella (R)	8th	223	CHOB	225-5341

MASSACHUSETTS
Senators
Name Party	Dist.	Room	Bldg.	Tele.
Edward M. Kennedy (D)		315	SROB	224-4543
John Kerry (D)		421	SROB	224-2742

Representatives
Name Party	Dist.	Room	Bldg.	Tele.
John W. Oliver (D)	1st	1323	LHOB	225-5335
Richard E. Neal (D)	2nd	131	CHOB	225-5601
Peter I. Blute (R)	3rd	1029	LHOB	225-6101
Barney Frank (D)	4th	2404	RHOB	225-5931
Martin T. Meehan (D)	5th	1216	LHOB	225-3411
Peter G. Torkildsen (R)	6th	120	CHOB	225-8020
Edward J. Markey (D)	7th	2133	RHOB	225-2836

Name Party	Dist.	Room	Bldg.	Tele.
Joseph P. Kennedy II (D)	8th	1210	LHOB	225-5111
Joe Moakley (D)	9th	235	CHOB	225-8273
Gerry E. Studds (D)	10th	237	CHOB	225-3111
MICHIGAN				
Senators				
Donald W. Riegle, Jr. (D)		105	DOB	224-4822
Carl Levin (D)		459	SROB	224-6221
Representatives				
Bart Stupak (D)	1st	317	CHOB	225-4735
Peter Hoekstra (R)	2nd	1319	LHOB	225-4401
Paul B. Henry (R)	3rd	1526	LHOB	225-3831
Dave Camp (R)	4th	137	CHOB	225-3561
James A. Barcia (D)	5th	1719	LHOB	225-8171
Fred Upton (R)	6th	2439	RHOB	225-3761
Nick Smith (R)	7th	1708	LHOB	225-6276
Bob Carr (D)	8th	2347	RHOB	225-4872
Dale E. Kildee (D)	9th	2239	RHOB	225-3611
David E. Bonior (D)	10th	2207	RHOB	225-2106
Joe Knollenberg (R)	11th	1218	LHOB	225-4735
Sander M. Levin (D)	12th	106	CHOB	225-4961
William D. Ford (D)	13th	2107	RHOB	225-6261
John Conyers, Jr. (D)	14th	2426	RHOB	225-5126
Barbara-Rose Collins (D)	15th	1108	LHOB	225-2261
John D. Dingell (D)	16th	2328	RHOB	225-4071
MINNESOTA				
Senators				
Dave Durenberger (R)		154	SROB	224-3244
Paul Wellstone (D)		702	SHOB	224-5641
Representatives				
Timothy J. Penny (D)	1st	436	CHOB	225-2472
David Minge (D)	2nd	1508	LHOB	225-2331
Jim Ramstad (R)	3rd	322	CHOB	225-2871
Bruce F. Vento (D)	4th	2304	RHOB	225-6631
Martin Olav Sabo (D)	5th	2336	RHOB	225-4755
Rod Grams (R)	6th	1713	LHOB	225-2271
Collin C. Peterson (D)	7th	1133	LHOB	225-2165
James L. Oberstar (D)	8th	2366	RHOB	225-6211
MISSISSIPPI				
Senators				
Thad Cochran (R)		326	SROB	224-5054
Trent Lott (R)		487	SROB	224-6253
Representatives				
Jamie L. Whitten (D)	1st	2314	RHOB	225-4306
Mike Espy (D)	2nd	2463	RHOB	225-5876
G.V. "Sonny" Montgomery (D)	3rd	2184	RHOB	225-5031
Mike Parker (D)	4th	1410	LHOB	225-5865
Gene Taylor (D)	5th	215	CHOB	225-5772
MISSOURI				
Senators				
John C. Danforth (R)		249	SROB	224-6154
Christopher S. Bond (R)		293	SROB	224-5721

Name Party	Dist.	Room	Bldg.	Tele.
Representatives				
William L. Clay (D)	1st	2306	RHOB	225-2406
James M. Talent (R)	2nd	1022	LHOB	225-2561
Richard A. Gephardt (D)	3rd	1432	LHOB	225-2671
Ike Skelton (D)	4th	2227	RHOB	225-2876
Alan Wheat (D)	5th	2334	RHOB	225-4535
Pat Danner (D)	6th	1217	LHOB	225-7041
Mel Hancock (R)	7th	1024	LHOB	225-6536
Bill Emerson (R)	8th	2454	RHOB	225-4404
Harold L. Volkmer (D)	9th	2409	RHOB	225-2956
MONTANA				
Senators				
Max Baucus (D)		706	SHOB	224-2651
Conrad Burns (R)		183	DOB	224-2644
Representative				
Pat Williams (D)	AL	2457	RHOB	225-3211
NEBRASKA				
Senators				
Jim Exon (D)		528	SHOB	224-4224
Bob Kerrey (D)		316	SHOB	224-6551
Representatives				
Doug Bereuter (R)	1st	2348	RHOB	225-4806
Peter Hoagland (D)	2nd	1113	LHOB	225-4155
Bill Barrett (R)	3rd	1213	LHOB	225-6435
NEVADA				
Senators				
Harry Reid (D)		324	SHOB	224-3542
Richard H. Bryan (D)		364	SROB	224-6244
Representatives				
James Bilbray (D)	1st	2431	RHOB	225-5965
Barbara F. Vucanovich (R)	2nd	2202	RHOB	225-6155
NEW HAMPSHIRE				
Senators				
Robert C. Smith (R)		332	DOB	224-2841
Judd Gregg (R)		513	SHOB	224-3324
Representatives				
Bill Zeliff (R)	1st	224	CHOB	225-5456
Dick Swett (D)	2nd	230	CHOB	225-5206
NEW JERSEY				
Senators				
Bill Bradley (D)		731	SHOB	224-3224
Frank R. Lautenberg (D)		506	SHOB	224-4744
Representatives				
Robert E. Andrews (D)	1st	1005	LHOB	225-6501
William J. Hughes (D)	2nd	241	CHOB	225-6572
H. James Saxton (R)	3rd	324	CHOB	225-4765
Christopher H. Smith (R)	4th	2353	RHOB	225-3765
Marge Roukema (R)	5th	2244	RHOB	225-4465
Frank Pallone, Jr. (D)	6th	420	CHOB	225-4671
Bob Franks (R)	7th	429	CHOB	225-5361

Name Party	Dist.	Room	Bldg.	Tele.
Herbert C. Klein (D)	8th	1728	LHOB	225-5751
Robert G. Torricelli (D)	9th	2159	RHOB	225-5061
Donald M. Payne (D)	10th	417	CHOB	225-3436
Dean A. Gallo (R)	11th	2447	RHOB	225-5034
Dick Zimmer (R)	12th	228	CHOB	225-5801
Robert Menendez (D)	13th	1531	LHOB	225-7919

NEW MEXICO
Senators

Name Party	Dist.	Room	Bldg.	Tele.
Pete V. Domenici (R)		427	DOB	224-6621
Jeff Bingaman (D)		524	SHOB	224-5521

Representatives

Name Party	Dist.	Room	Bldg.	Tele.
Steven H. Schiff (R)	1st	1009	LHOB	225-6316
Joe Skeen (R)	2nd	2367	RHOB	225-2365
Bill Richardson (D)	3rd	2349	RHOB	225-6190

NEW YORK
Senators

Name Party	Dist.	Room	Bldg.	Tele.
Daniel Patrick Moynihan (D)		464	SROB	224-4451
Alfonse M. D'Amato (R)		520	SHOB	224-6542

Representatives

Name Party	Dist.	Room	Bldg.	Tele.
George J. Hochbrueckner (D)	1st	229	CHOB	225-3826
Rick A. Lazio (R)	2nd	314	CHOB	225-3335
Peter T. King (R)	3rd	118	CHOB	225-7896
David A. Levy (R)	4th	116	CHOB	225-5516
Gary L. Ackerman (D)	5th	238	CHOB	225-2601
Floyd H. Flake (D)	6th	1035	LHOB	225-3461
Thomas J. Manton (D)	7th	203	CHOB	225-3965
Jerrold Nadler (D)	8th	424	CHOB	225-5635
Charles E. Schumer (D)	9th	2412	RHOB	225-6616
Edolphus Towns (D)	10th	2232	RHOB	225-5936
Major R. Owens (D)	11th	2305	RHOB	225-6231
Nydia M. Velazquez (D)	12th	132	CHOB	225-2361
Susan Molinari (R)	13th	123	CHOB	225-3371
Carolyn B. Maloney (D)	14th	1504	LHOB	225-7944
Charles B. Rangel (D)	15th	2252	RHOB	225-4365
Jose E. Serrano (D)	16th	336	CHOB	225-4361
Eliot L. Engel (D)	17th	1434	LHOB	225-2464
Nita M. Lowey (D)	18th	1424	LHOB	225-6506
Hamilton Fish, Jr. (R)	19th	2354	RHOB	225-5441
Benjamin A. Gilman (R)	20th	2185	RHOB	225-3776
Michael R. McNulty (D)	21st	217	CHOB	225-5076
Gerald B.H. Solomon (R)	22nd	2265	RHOB	225-5614
Sherwood Boehlert (R)	23rd	1127	LHOB	225-3665
John M. McHugh (R)	24th	416	CHOB	225-4611
James T. Walsh (R)	25th	1330	LHOB	225-3701
Maurice D. Hinchey (D)	26th	1313	LHOB	225-6335
Bill Paxon (R)	27th	1314	LHOB	225-5265
Louise M. Slaughter (D)	28th	2421	RHOB	225-3615
John J. LaFalce (D)	29th	2310	RHOB	225-3231
Jack Quinn (R)	30th	331	CHOB	225-3306
Amo Houghton (R)	31st	1110	LHOB	225-3161

NORTH CAROLINA
Senators

Name Party	Dist.	Room	Bldg.	Tele.
Jesse Helms (R)		403	DOB	224-6342
Lauch Faircloth (R)		716	SHOB	224-3154

Representatives

Name Party	Dist.	Room	Bldg.	Tele.
Eva Clayton (D)	1st	222	CHOB	225-3101
Tim Valentine (D)	2nd	2229	RHOB	225-4531
H. Martin Lancaster (D)	3rd	2436	RHOB	225-3415
David Price (D)	4th	2458	RHOB	225-1784
Stephen L. Neal (D)	5th	2469	RHOB	225-2071
Howard Coble (R)	6th	403	CHOB	225-3065
Charlie Rose (D)	7th	2230	RHOB	225-2731
W.G. "Bill" Hefner (D)	8th	2470	RHOB	225-3715
Alex McMillan (R)	9th	401	CHOB	225-1976
Cass Ballenger (R)	10th	2238	RHOB	225-2576
Charles H. Taylor (R)	11th	516	CHOB	225-6401
Melvin Watt (D)	12th	1232	LHOB	225-1510

NORTH DAKOTA
Senators

Name Party	Dist.	Room	Bldg.	Tele.
Kent Conrad (D)		724	SHOB	224-2043
Byron L. Dorgan (D)		825	SHOB	224-2551

Representative

Name Party	Dist.	Room	Bldg.	Tele.
Earl Pomeroy (D)	AL	318	CHOB	225-2611

OHIO
Senators

Name Party	Dist.	Room	Bldg.	Tele.
John Glenn (D)		503	SHOB	224-3353
Howard M. Metzenbaum (D)		140	SROB	224-2315

Representatives

Name Party	Dist.	Room	Bldg.	Tele.
David Mann (D)	1st	503	CHOB	225-2216
Bill Gradison (R)	2nd	1536	LHOB	225-3164
Tony P. Hall (D)	3rd	2264	RHOB	225-6465
Michael G. Oxley (R)	4th	2233	RHOB	225-2676
Paul E. Gillmor (R)	5th	1203	LHOB	225-6405
Ted Strickland (D)	6th	1429	LHOB	225-5705
David L. Hobson (R)	7th	1507	LHOB	225-4324
John A. Boehner (R)	8th	1020	LHOB	225-6205
Marcy Kaptur (D)	9th	2104	RHOB	225-4146
Martin R. Hoke (R)	10th	212	CHOB	225-5871
Louis Stokes (D)	11th	2365	RHOB	225-7032
John R. Kasich (R)	12th	1131	LHOB	225-5355
Sherrod Brown (D)	13th	1407	LHOB	225-3401
Tom Sawyer (D)	14th	1414	LHOB	225-5231
Deborah Pryce (R)	15th	128	CHOB	225-2015
Ralph Regula (R)	16th	2309	RHOB	225-3876
James A. Traficant, Jr. (D)	17th	2446	RHOB	225-5261
Douglas Applegate (D)	18th	2183	RHOB	225-6265
Eric D. Fingerhut (D)	19th	431	CHOB	225-5731

OKLAHOMA
Senators

Name Party	Dist.	Room	Bldg.	Tele.
David L. Boren (D)		453	SROB	224-4721
Don Nickles (R)		713	SHOB	224-5754

Name Party	Dist.	Room	Bldg.	Tele.
Representatives				
James M. Inhofe (R)	1st	442	CHOB	225-2211
Mike Synar (D)	2nd	2329	RHOB	225-2701
Bill Brewster (D)	3rd	1727	LHOB	225-4565
Dave McCurdy (D)	4th	2344	RHOB	225-6165
Ernest Jim Istook (R)	5th	1116	LHOB	225-2132
Glenn English (D)	6th	2206	RHOB	225-5565
OREGON				
Senators				
Mark O. Hatfield (R)		711	SHOB	224-3753
Bob Packwood (R)		259	SROB	224-5244
Representatives				
Elizabeth Furse (D)	1st	316	CHOB	225-0855
Bob Smith (R)	2nd	108	CHOB	225-6730
Ron Wyden (D)	3rd	1111	LHOB	225-4811
Peter A. DeFazio (D)	4th	1233	LHOB	225-6416
Mike Kopetski (D)	5th	218	CHOB	225-5711
PENNSYLVANIA				
Senators				
Arlen Specter (R)		303	SHOB	224-4254
Harris Wofford (D)		283	SROB	224-6324
Representatives				
Thomas M. Foglietta (D)	1st	341	CHOB	225-4731
Lucien E. Blackwell (D)	2nd	410	CHOB	225-4001
Robert A. Borski (D)	3rd	2161	RHOB	225-8251
Ron Klink (D)	4th	1130	LHOB	225-2565
William F. Clinger (R)	5th	2160	RHOB	225-5121
Tim Holden (D)	6th	1421	LHOB	225-5546
Curt Weldon (R)	7th	2452	RHOB	225-2011
Jim Greenwood (R)	8th	515	CHOB	225-4276
Bud Shuster (R)	9th	2188	RHOB	225-2431
Joseph M. McDade (R)	10th	2370	RHOB	225-3731
Paul E. Kanjorski (D)	11th	2429	RHOB	225-6511
John P. Murtha (D)	12th	2423	RHOB	225-2065
Marjorie Margolies-Mezvinsky (D)	13th	1516	LHOB	225-6111
William J. Coyne (D)	14th	2455	RHOB	225-2301
Paul McHale (D)	15th	511	CHOB	225-6411
Robert S. Walker (R)	16th	2369	RHOB	225-2411
George W. Gekas (R)	17th	2410	RHOB	225-4315
Rick Santorum (R)	18th	1222	LHOB	225-2135
Bill Goodling (R)	19th	2263	RHOB	225-5836
Austin J. Murphy (D)	20th	2210	RHOB	225-4665
Tom Ridge (R)	21st	1714	LHOB	225-5406
PUERTO RICO				
Representative				
Carlos Romero-Barcelo (D)	AL	1517	LHOB	225-2615
RHODE ISLAND				
Senators				
Claiborne Pell (D)		335	SROB	224-4642
John H. Chafee (R)		567	DOB	224-2921

Name Party	Dist.	Room	Bldg.	Tele.
Representatives				
Ronald K. Machtley (R)	1st	326	CHOB	225-4911
Jack Reed (D)	2nd	1510	LHOB	225-2735
SOUTH CAROLINA				
Senators				
Strom Thurmond (R)		217	SROB	224-5972
Ernest F. Hollings (D)		125	SROB	224-6121
Representatives				
Arthur Ravenel, Jr. (R)	1st	231	CHOB	225-3176
Floyd D. Spence (R)	2nd	2405	RHOB	225-2452
Butler Derrick (D)	3rd	221	CHOB	225-5301
Bob Inglis (R)	4th	1237	LHOB	225-6030
John M. Spratt, Jr. (D)	5th	1533	LHOB	225-5501
James E. Clayburn (D)	6th	319	CHOB	225-3315
SOUTH DAKOTA				
Senators				
Larry Pressler (R)		133	SHOB	224-5842
Tom Daschle (D)		317	SHOB	224-2321
Representative				
Tim Johnson (D)	AL	2438	RHOB	225-2801
TENNESSEE				
Senators				
Jim Sasser (D)		363	SROB	224-3344
Harlan Mathews (D)		505	DOB	224-1036
Representatives				
James H. Quillen (R)	1st	102	CHOB	225-6356
John J. "Jimmy" Duncan, Jr. (R)	2nd	115	CHOB	225-5435
Marilyn Lloyd (D)	3rd	2406	RHOB	225-3271
Jim Cooper (D)	4th	125	CHOB	225-6831
Bob Clement (D)	5th	1230	LHOB	225-4311
Bart Gordon (D)	6th	103	CHOB	225-4231
Don Sundquist (R)	7th	438	CHOB	225-2811
John Tanner (D)	8th	1427	LHOB	225-4714
Harold E. Ford (D)	9th	2211	RHOB	225-3265
TEXAS				
Senators				
Bob Krueger* (D)		703	SHOB	224-5922
Phil Gramm (R)		370	SROB	224-2934

*Seat vacated by Lloyd Bentsen when he became secretary of treasury. Permanent replacement to be determined in May 1993 election.

Name Party	Dist.	Room	Bldg.	Tele.
Representatives				
Jim Chapman (D)	1st	2417	RHOB	225-3035
Charles Wilson (D)	2nd	2256	RHOB	225-2401
Sam Johnson (R)	3rd	1030	LHOB	225-4201
Ralph M. Hall (D)	4th	2236	RHOB	225-6673
John Bryant (D)	5th	205	CHOB	225-2231
Joe L. Barton (R)	6th	1514	LHOB	225-2002
Bill Archer (R)	7th	1236	LHOB	225-2571
Jack Fields (R)	8th	2228	RHOB	225-4901
Jack Brooks (D)	9th	2449	RHOB	225-6565

Name Party	Dist.	Room	Bldg.	Tele.
J.J. Pickle (D)	10th	242	CHOB	225-4865
Chet Edwards (D)	11th	328	CHOB	225-6105
Pete Geren (D)	12th	1730	LHOB	225-5071
Bill Sarpalius (D)	13th	126	CHOB	225-3706
Greg Laughlin (D)	14th	236	CHOB	225-2831
E. "Kika" de la Garza (D)	15th	1401	LHOB	225-2531
Ronald D. Coleman (D)	16th	440	CHOB	225-4831
Charles W. Stenholm (D)	17th	1211	LHOB	225-6605
Craig Washington (D)	18th	1711	LHOB	225-3816
Larry Combest (R)	19th	1511	LHOB	225-4005
Henry B. Gonzalez (D)	20th	2413	RHOB	225-3236
Lamar Smith (R)	21st	2443	RHOB	225-4236
Tom DeLay (R)	22nd	407	CHOB	225-5951
Henry Bonilla (R)	23rd	1529	LHOB	225-4511
Martin Frost (D)	24th	2459	RHOB	225-3605
Michael A. Andrews (D)	25th	303	CHOB	225-7508
Dick Armey (R)	26th	301	CHOB	225-7772
Solomon P. Ortiz (D)	27th	2445	RHOB	225-7742
Frank Tejeda (D)	28th	323	CHOB	225-1640
Gene Green (D)	29th	1004	LHOB	225-1688
Eddie Bernice Johnson (D)	30th	1721	LHOB	225-8885

UTAH
Senators

Name Party	Dist.	Room	Bldg.	Tele.
Orrin G. Hatch (R)		135	SROB	224-5251
Robert F. Bennett (R)		B40	DOB	224-5444

Representatives

Name Party	Dist.	Room	Bldg.	Tele.
James V. Hansen (R)	1st	2466	RHOB	225-0453
Karen Shepherd (D)	2nd	414	CHOB	225-3011
Bill Orton (D)	3rd	1122	LHOB	225-7751

VERMONT
Senators

Name Party	Dist.	Room	Bldg.	Tele.
Patrick J. Leahy (D)		433	SROB	224-4242
James M. Jeffords (R)		530	DOB	224-5141

Representative

Name Party	Dist.	Room	Bldg.	Tele.
Bernard Sanders (Independent)	AL	213	CHOB	225-4115

VIRGIN ISLANDS
Representative

Name Party	Dist.	Room	Bldg.	Tele.
Ron de Lugo (D)	AL	2427	RHOB	225-1790

VIRGINIA
Senators

Name Party	Dist.	Room	Bldg.	Tele.
John W. Warner (R)		225	SROB	224-2023
Charles S. Robb (D)		493	SROB	224-4024

Representatives

Name Party	Dist.	Room	Bldg.	Tele.
Herbert H. Bateman (R)	1st	2350	RHOB	225-4261
Owen B. Pickett (D)	2nd	2430	RHOB	225-4215
Robert C. Scott (D)	3rd	501	CHOB	225-8351
Norman Sisisky (D)	4th	2352	RHOB	225-6365
Lewis F. Payne, Jr. (D)	5th	1119	LHOB	225-4711

Name Party	Dist.	Room	Bldg.	Tele.
Robert W. Goodlatte (R)	6th	214	CHOB	225-5431
Thomas J. Bliley, Jr. (R)	7th	2241	RHOB	225-2815
James P. Moran, Jr. (D)	8th	430	CHOB	225-4376
Rick Boucher (D)	9th	2245	RHOB	225-3861
Frank R. Wolf (R)	10th	104	CHOB	225-5136
Leslie L. Byrne (D)	11th	1609	LHOB	225-1492

WASHINGTON
Senators

Name Party	Dist.	Room	Bldg.	Tele.
Slade Gorton (R)		730	SHOB	224-3441
Patty Murray (D)		B34	DOB	224-2621

Representatives

Name Party	Dist.	Room	Bldg.	Tele.
Maria Cantwell (D)	1st	1520	LHOB	225-6311
Al Swift (D)	2nd	1502	LHOB	225-2605
Jolene Unsoeld (D)	3rd	1527	LHOB	225-3536
Jay Inslee (D)	4th	1431	LHOB	225-5816
Thomas S. Foley (D)	5th	1201	LHOB	225-2006
Norm Dicks (D)	6th	2467	RHOB	225-5916
Jim McDermott (D)	7th	1707	LHOB	225-3106
Jennifer Dunn (R)	8th	1641	LHOB	225-7761
Mike Kreidler (D)	9th	1535	LHOB	225-8901

WEST VIRGINIA
Senators

Name Party	Dist.	Room	Bldg.	Tele.
Robert C. Byrd (D)		311	SHOB	224-3954
John D. Rockefeller IV (D)		109	SHOB	224-6472

Representatives

Name Party	Dist.	Room	Bldg.	Tele.
Alan B. Mollohan (D)	1st	2242	RHOB	225-4172
Bob Wise (D)	2nd	2434	RHOB	225-2711
Nick J. Rahall II (D)	3rd	2269	RHOB	225-3452

WISCONSIN
Senators

Name Party	Dist.	Room	Bldg.	Tele.
Herb Kohl (D)		330	SHOB	224-5653
Russell D. Feingold (D)		B40	DOB	224-5323

Representatives

Name Party	Dist.	Room	Bldg.	Tele.
Les Aspin (D)	1st	2108	RHOB	225-3031
Scott L. Klug (R)	2nd	1224	LHOB	225-2906
Steve Gunderson (R)	3rd	2235	RHOB	225-5506
Gerald D. Kleczka (D)	4th	2301	RHOB	225-4572
Thomas M. Barrett (D)	5th	313	CHOB	225-3571
Tom Petri (R)	6th	2262	RHOB	225-2476
David R. Obey (D)	7th	2462	RHOB	225-3365
Toby Roth (R)	8th	2234	RHOB	225-5665
F. James Sensenbrenner, Jr. (R)	9th	2332	RHOB	225-5101

WYOMING
Senators

Name Party	Dist.	Room	Bldg.	Tele.
Malcolm Wallop (R)		237	SROB	224-6441
Alan K. Simpson (R)		261	DOB	224-3424

Representative

Name Party	Dist.	Room	Bldg.	Tele.
Craig Thomas (R)	AL	1019	LHOB	225-2311

Appendix 2

How to write to drug manufacturers

Following is a list of prominent drug companies operating in the United States that are members of the Pharmaceutical Manufacturers Association. Each listing includes an address and the name of a senior company executive.

Many of these companies have subsidiaries or marketing arms that are not listed below. The list is current as of February 1993.

Abbott Laboratories
One Abbott Park Rd.
Abbott Park, IL 60064
Chairman and CEO: Duane L. Burnham

Adria Laboratories
(Division of Erbamont Inc.)
P.O. Box 16529
Columbus, OH 43216
Acting President: Fernando da Costa

Alcon Laboratories Inc.
(Subsidiary of Nestle, S.A.)
6201 South Freeway
Fort Worth, TX 76134-2099
President: Edgar Schollmaier

Allergan Inc.
2525 Du Pont Drive
P.O. Box 19534
Irvine, CA 92713-9534
Chairman and CEO: Gavin S. Herbert

Altana Inc.
60 Baylis Road
Melville, NY 11747
President: Rolf Rahmstorf

Alza Corporation
950 Page Mill Road
P.O. Box 10950
Palo Alto, CA 94303
Co-chairman and CEO: Martin S. Gerstel

American Home Products Corporation
31st floor
685 Third Avenue
New York, NY 10017
Chairman and CEO: John R. Stafford

Amgen Inc.
Amgen Center
1840 DeHavilland Dr.
Thousand Oaks, CA 91320-1789
Chairman and CEO: Gordon M. Binder

Anaquest
(Subsidiary of BOC Health Care Inc.)
110 Allen Road
Box 804
Liberty Corner, NJ 07938-0804
President: Martin McGlynn

B.F. Ascher & Company Inc.
15501 West 109th Street
Lenexa, KS 66219
President: James S. Ascher

Astra Pharmaceutical Products Inc.
(Subsidiary of AB Astra)
50 Otis Street
Westborough, MA 01581
President: Lars Bildman

Berlex Laboratories Inc.
(Subsidiary of Schering AG)
300 Fairfield Road
Wayne, NJ 07470
President and CEO: Jorge Engel

Boehringer Ingelheim Corporation
(Part of Boehringer Ingelheim GmbH)
900 Ridgebury Road
P.O. Box 368
Ridgefield, CT 06877
President and CEO: Werner Gerstenberg

Boots Pharmaceuticals Inc.
(Subsidiary of The Boots Company PLC)
Suite 200
300 Tri-State International Center
Lincolnshire, IL 60069
President: Carter H. Eckert

Bristol-Myers Squibb Company
345 Park Avenue
New York, NY 10154
Chairman and CEO: Richard L. Gelb

Burroughs Wellcome Co.
(Subsidiary of Wellcome Foundation)
3030 Cornwallis Road
Research Triangle Park, NC 27709
President and CEO: Philip R. Tracy

Carter-Wallace Inc.
1345 Avenue of the Americas
New York, NY 10105
Chairman and CEO: Henry H. Hoyt, Jr.

Central Pharmaceuticals Inc.
120 East Third Street
Seymour, IN 47274
President and CEO: Daniel J. Desmond

Ciba-Geigy Corporation
(U.S. Pharmaceuticals Division)
556 Morris Avenue
Summit, NJ 07901
Division President: Douglas Watson

Connaught Laboratories Inc.
(Subsidiary of Connaught Labs Ltd.)
P.O. Box 187
Swiftwater, PA 18370
President: David J. Williams

The Du Pont Merck Pharmaceutical Co.
P.O. Box 80025
Wilmington, DE 19880-0025
President and CEO: Joseph A. Mollica

Ferndale Laboratories Inc.
780 West Eight Mile Road
Ferndale, MI 48220
President: David Beens

Fisons Corporation
(Part of Fisons PLC)
755 Jefferson Road
P.O. Box 1710
Rochester, NY 14603
President: Heimo Reulecke

Genentech Inc.
460 Point San Bruno Boulevard
South San Francisco, CA 94080
President and CEO: Kirk Raab

Glaxo Inc.
(Subsidiary of Glaxo Holdings PLC)
Five Moore Drive
Box 13398
Research Triangle Park, NC 27709
Chairman and CEO: Charles Sanders

Gynopharma Inc.
50 Division Street
Somerville, NJ 08876
CEO: Rod Mackenzie

Hoechst–Roussel Pharmaceuticals Inc.
(Affiliate of Hoechst AG)
Route 202–206
P.O. Box 2500
Somerville, NJ 08876-1258
President: Jack Herdklotz

Hoffmann–La Roche Inc.
(Subsidiary of Roche Holdings)
340 Kingsland Street
Nutley, NJ 07110
President and CEO: Patrick Zenner

ICI Pharmaceuticals Group
(Business unit of ICI Americas Inc.)
Wilmington, DE 19897
President (of U.S. pharmaceutical unit of ICI PLC):
   Robert C. Black

Janssen Pharmaceutica Inc.
(Subsidiary of Johnson & Johnson)
1125 Trenton-Harbourton Road
P.O. Box 200
Titusville, NJ 08560-0200
President: Larry Pickering

Johnson & Johnson
One Johnson & Johnson Plaza
New Brunswick, NJ 08933-7204
Chairman and CEO: Ralph S. Larsen

Kabi Pharmacia Inc.
(Division of Procordia, U.S.)
800 Centennial Avenue
Piscataway, NJ 08855-1327
President: Anders Wiklund

Knoll Pharmaceutical Company
(Subsidiary of BASF Corp.)
30 North Jefferson Road
Whippany, NJ 07981
President: Gerald Bendele

Lederle Laboratories
(Division of American Cyanamid Company)
One Cyanamid Plaza
Wayne, NJ 07470
President: Edward Fritzky

Eli Lilly and Company
Lilly Corporate Center
Indianapolis, IN 46285
President: Vaughn Bryson

Marion Merrell Dow Inc.
9300 Ward Parkway
P.O. Box 8480
Kansas City, MO 46114
President and CEO: Fred W. Lyons, Jr.

McNeil Pharmaceutical
(Subsidiary of Johnson & Johnson)
Welsh & McKean Roads
Spring House, PA 19477-0776
President: Michael D. Casey

Merck & Co. Inc.
One Merck Drive
P.O. Box 100
Whitehouse Station, NJ 08889-0100
Chairman and CEO: P. Roy Vagelos

Miles Inc.
(Subsidiary of Bayer AG)
One Mellon Center
500 Grant Street
Pittsburgh, PA 15219-2502
President and CEO: Helge H. Wehmeier

Organon Inc.
(Affiliate of Akzo Pharma BV)
375 Mt. Pleasant Avenue
West Orange, NJ 07052
President: Brian Haigh

Parke-Davis
(Division of Warner-Lambert Company)
201 Tabor Road
Morris Plains, NJ 07950
President: Joseph Smith

Pfizer Inc.
235 East 42nd Street
New York, NY 10017
Chairman and CEO: William C. Steere

The Procter & Gamble Company
One Procter & Gamble Plaza
Cincinnati, OH 45202
Chairman and CEO: Edwin L. Artzt

The Purdue Frederick Company
100 Connecticut Avenue
Norwalk, CT 06856
President: Dr. Raymond Sackler

Reed & Carnrick
(Division of Block Drug Company)
257 Cornelison Ave.
Jersey City, NJ 07302
President: John T. Spitznagel

Rhône-Poulenc Rorer Inc.
500 Arcola Road
P.O. Box 1200
Collegeville, PA 19426-0107
Chairman and CEO: Robert Cawthorn

Sandoz Pharmaceuticals Corporation
(Subsidiary of Sandoz Ltd.)
59 Route 10
East Hanover, NJ 07936
President and CEO: Timothy Rothwell

Schering-Plough Corporation
One Giralda Farms
Madison, NJ 07940-1000
President and CEO: Richard Kogan

Schwarz Pharma
(Subsidiary of Schwarz Pharma, AG)
5600 West County Line Road
Mequon, WI 53092
President: J.A. Troup

Searle
(Subsidiary of Monsanto Co.)
P.O. Box 5110
Chicago, IL 60680
CEO: Sheldon Gilgore

SmithKline Beecham
U.S. headquarters:
One Franklin Plaza
P.O. Box 7929
Philadelphia, PA 19101
President and CEO: Robert Bauman

Solvay Pharmaceuticals
(Subsidiary of Solvay SA)
901 Sawyer Road
Marietta, GA 30062
President and CEO: Dr. James Warren

Sterling Winthrop Inc.
(Subsidiary of Eastman Kodak Co.)
90 Park Ave.
New York, NY 10016
CEO: Louis P. Mattis

Syntex Corp.
3401 Hillview Ave.
Palo Alto, CA 94304
CEO: Paul Freiman

The Upjohn Co.
7000 Portage Road
Kalamazoo, MI 49001
CEO: Dr. Theodore Cooper

Warner-Lambert Company
201 Tabor Road
Morris Plains, NJ 07950
CEO and Chairman: Melvin R. Goodes

Wyeth-Ayerst Laboratories
(Division of American Home Products Corporation)
555 E. Lancaster Ave.
St. Davids, PA 19087
President: Fred Hassan

Appendix 3

The most prescribed drugs in America

Following is a list of the two hundred drugs most frequently dispensed by American pharmacies in 1991. They are listed in alphabetical order by trade name. If it's a generic drug, it is listed by its chemical name and is followed by an asterisk.

Four pieces of information follow the drug name: a number indicating its ranking on the list of two hundred most frequently filled prescriptions; the drug's manufacturer; a key medical indication for which the drug is generally prescribed; and either the drug's chemical name (if it is a brand-name product) or the drug's brand-name version (if it is a generic medicine).

The information was prepared by Stephen H. Paul, chairman of pharmaceutical economics and health care delivery at Temple University School of Pharmacy in Philadelphia. The rankings are from the magazine *Pharmacy Times*.

Some manufacturers' names are followed by a second name in parentheses; the second name represents the division of the manufacturer associated with the drug.

Drug	Rank	Manufacturer	Purpose	Chemical or Brand Name
Amoxicillin trihydrate*	33	Biocraft	Infection	Generic version of Amoxil; Polymox; Trimox; Wymox
Amoxicillin trihydrate*	54	Warner-Lambert (Warner Chilcott)	Infection	Generic version of Amoxil; Polymox; Trimox; Wymox
Amoxil	1	SmithKline Beecham	Infection	Amoxicillin trihydrate
Anaprox DS	58	Syntex	Arthritis; pain	Naproxen sodium
Ansaid	77	Upjohn	Arthritis; pain	Flurbiprofen
Ativan	91	American Home Products (Wyeth-Ayerst)	Anxiety	Lorazepam
Atrovent	85	Boehringer Ingelheim	Asthma	Ipratropium bromide
Augmentin	18	SmithKline Beecham	Infection	Amoxicillin and potassium clavulante
Axid	115	Eli Lilly	Ulcers	Nizatidine
Azmacort	154	Rhône-Poulenc Rorer	Asthma	Triamcinolone acetonide
Bactroban	125	SmithKline Beecham	Infection	Mupirocin
Beconase-AQ	89	Glaxo (Allen & Hanburys)	Asthma	Beclomethasone dipropionate
Beepen-VK	174	SmithKline Beecham	Infection	Penicillin V potassium
Bumex	110	Roche Laboratories	Cardiovascular disease	Bumetanide
Buspar	82	Bristol Myers-Squibb (Mead Johnson)	Anxiety	Buspirone
Calan SR	16	Searle	Cardiovascular disease	Verapamil
Capoten	14	Bristol Myers-Squibb (Squibb)	Cardiovascular disease	Captopril
Carafate	68	Marion Merrell Dow	Ulcers	Sucralfate
Cardizem	17	Marion Merrell Dow	Cardiovascular disease	Diltiazem
Cardizem SR	42	Marion Merrell Dow	Cardiovascular disease	Diltiazem
Ceclor	7	Eli Lilly	Infection	Cefaclor
Ceftin	56	Glaxo (Allen & Hanburys)	Infection	Cefuroxime
Cephalexin*	83	Biocraft	Infection	Generic version of Keflex
Cephalexin*	146	Bristol-Myers Squibb (Apothecon)	Infection	Generic version of Keflex
Cipro	27	Miles Inc.	Infection	Ciprofloxacin
Cleocin T	158	Upjohn	Acne	Clindamycin, topical
Clinoril	198	Merck (MS&D)	Arthritis; pain	Sulindac
Codeine phosphate and acetaminophen*	57	Purepac	Pain	Generic version of Tylenol with codeine

Drug	Rank	Manufacturer	Purpose	Chemical or Brand Name
Codeine phosphate and acetaminophen*	100	Barr	Pain	Generic version of Tylenol with codeine
Codeine phosphate and acetaminophen*	105	Lemmon Co.	Pain	Generic version of Tylenol with codeine
Codeine phosphate and acetaminophen*	150	Rugby Labs	Pain	Generic version of Tylenol with codeine
Codeine phosphate and acetaminophen*	167	Halsey Drug Co.	Pain	Generic version of Tylenol with codeine
Compazine	159	SmithKline Beecham	Anxiety	Prochlorperazine
Corgard	81	Bristol Myers-Squibb (Bristol Labs)	Cardiovascular disease	Nadolol
Coumadin Sodium	37	Du Pont Merck Pharmaceutical	Blood clots	Warfarin sodium
Cyclobenzaprine HCl*	139	Danbury Pharmacal	Muscle spasm	Generic version of Flexeril
Darvocet-N 100	32	Eli Lilly	Arthritis; pain	Propoxyphene napsylate and acetaminophen
Deltasone	138	Upjohn	Inflammation	Prednisone
Demulen 1/35-28	161	Searle	Contraception	Ethinyl estradiol and ethynodiol diacetate
Depakote	194	Abbott Laboratories	Epilepsy	Divalproex sodium
Diabeta	43	Hoechst-Roussel	Diabetes	Glyburide
Diazepam*	182	Mylan Pharmaceuticals	Anxiety	Generic version of Valium
Dilantin	24	Warner-Lambert (Parke Davis)	Epilepsy	Phenytoin
Dipyridamole*	163	Barr Laboratories	Blood clots	Generic version of Persantine
Dolobid	131	Merck (MS&D)	Pain	Diflunisal
Donnatal	178	American Home Products (Wyeth-Ayerst)	Stomach cramps	Atropine and scopolamine and hyoscyamine
Duricef	50	Bristol Myers-Squibb (Mead Johnson)	Infection	Cefadroxil
Dyazide	13	SmithKline Beecham	Cardiovascular disease	Triamterene and hydrochlorthiazide
E.E.S.	87	Abbott	Infection	Erythromycin ethylsuccinate
Elavil	180	ICI Americas (Stuart)	Depression	Amitriptyline
E-Mycin 333	107	Boots Laboratories	Infection	Erythromycin
Entex LA	80	Proctor & Gamble	Cough	Phenylpropanolomine and guaifenesin
Eryc	124	Warner-Lambert (Parke Davis)	Infection	Erythromycin base
Ery-tab	133	Abbott	Infection	Erythromycin
Erythrocin Stearate	144	Abbott	Infection	Erythromycin stearate
Estrace oral	171	Bristol Myers-Squibb (Mead Johnson)	Menopause symptoms	Estradiol
Estraderm	55	Ciba-Geigy	Menopause symptoms	Estradiol transdermal system
Feldene	45	Pfizer	Arthritis; pain	Piroxicam
Fioricet	197	Sandoz	Migraine	Butalbital and acetaminophen and caffeine
Fiorinal	166	Sandoz	Migraine	Butalbital and aspirin and caffeine
Fiorinal/Codeine	132	Sandoz	Migraine	Butalbital and aspirin and caffeine and codeine
Flexeril	140	Merck (MS&D)	Muscle spasm	Cyclobenzaprine
Furosemide*	108	Rugby Labs	Cardiovascular disease	Generic version of Lasix
Furosemide*	114	Ciba-Geigy (Geneva Chemicals)	Cardiovascular disease	Generic version of Lasix
Furosemide*	120	Lederle	Cardiovascular disease	Generic version of Lasix
Furosemide*	137	Mylan	Cardiovascular disease	Generic version of Lasix
Glucotrol	44	Pfizer (Roerig)	Diabetes	Glipizide
Halcion	38	Upjohn	Insomnia	Triazolam
Hismanal	47	Johnson & Johnson (Janssen)	Allergy	Astemizole
Humulin N	34	Eli Lilly	Diabetes	Isophane insulin suspension
Humulin R	157	Eli Lilly	Diabetes	Insulin injection
Hydrochlorothiazide*	135	Rugby Labs	Cardiovascular disease	Generic version of Hydro-Diuril, Esidrex, and Oretic
Hydrocodone and acetaminophen*	63	Barr	Pain	Generic version of Lortab and Vicodin
Hytrin	86	Abbott	Cardiovascular disease	Terazosin
Ibuprofen*	41	Boots Pharmaceuticals	Arthritis; pain	Generic version of Motrin
Ibuprofen*	175	Rugby Labs	Arthritis; pain	Generic version of Motrin
Iletin I NPH	109	Eli Lilly	Diabetes	Isophane insulin suspension

Drug	Rank	Manufacturer	Purpose	Chemical or Brand Name
Inderal	88	American Home Products (Wyeth-Ayerst)	Cardiovascular disease, migraine	Propranolol
Inderal LA	101	American Home Products (Wyeth-Ayerst)	Cardiovascular disease, migraine	Propranolol
Intal	130	Fisons	Asthma	Cromolyn sodium
Iodinated glycerol and dextromethorphan*	200	Barre	Cough	Generic version of Tussi-Organidin DM
Isoptin SR	121	Knoll	Cardiovascular disease	Verapamil
Isordil	148	American Home Products (Wyeth-Ayerst)	Chest pain	Isosorbide dinitrate, oral
K-Dur	67	Schering-Plough (Key)	Potassium deficiency	Potassium chloride
Keflex	177	Eli Lilly (Dista)	Infection	Cephalexin
Keftab	186	Eli Lilly (Dista)	Infection	Cephalexin HCl monohydrate
Klonopin	98	Roche Laboratories	Epilepsy	Clonazepam
K-Tabs	151	Abbott	Potassium deficiency	Potassium chloride
Lanoxin	4	Burroughs Wellcome	Abnormal heart rhythm	Digoxin
Lasix	29	Hoechst-Roussel	Cardiovascular disease	Furosemide
Lo/Ovral-21	181	American Home Products (Wyeth-Ayerst)	Contraception	Ethinyl estradiol and norgestrel
Lo/Ovral-28	84	American Home Products (Wyeth-Ayerst)	Contraception	Ethinyl estradiol and norgestrel
Lodine	172	American Home Products (Wyeth-Ayerst)	Arthritis	Etodolac
Lopid	39	Warner-Lambert (Parke Davis)	High cholesterol	Gemfibrozil
Lopressor	23	Ciba-Geigy (Geigy)	Cardiovascular disease	Metoprolol tartrate
Lorazepam*	196	Purepac	Anxiety	Generic version of Ativan
Lorcet Plus	173	UAD Labs	Pain	Hydrocodone acetaminophen
Lortab 7.5/500	113	Whitby	Pain	Hydrocodone acetaminophen
Lotrimin	183	Schering-Plough	Infection	Clotrimazole
Lotrisone	66	Schering-Plough	Rash and fungus	Betamathosone and clotrimazole
Lozol	69	Rhône-Poulenc Rorer	Cardiovascular disease	Indapamide
Macrodantin	74	Procter & Gamble	Infection	Nitrofurantoin macrocrystals
Maxzide	111	Lederle	Cardiovascular disease	Triamterene and hydrochlorthiazide
Maxzide-25	122	Lederle	Cardiovascular disease	Triamterene and hydrochlorthiazide
Mevacor	21	Merck (MS&D)	High cholesterol	Lovastatin
Micro-K 10	78	American Home Products (Wyeth-Ayerst)	Potassium deficiency	Potassium chloride
Micronase	26	Upjohn	Diabetes	Glyburide
Monistat-7	192	Johnson & Johnson (Ortho ACP)	Infection	Miconazole
Motrin	70	Upjohn	Pain	Ibuprofen
Naprosyn	12	Syntex	Arthritis; pain	Naproxen
Nicorette	90	Marion Merrell Dow	Smoking	Nicotine polacrilex
Nitro-Dur	116	Schering-Plough (Key)	Heart pain	Nitroglycerine
Nitrostat	53	Warner-Lambert (Parke Davis)	Heart pain	Nitroglycerine
Nolvadex	129	ICI Americas	Cancer	Tamoxifen citrate
Nordette-28	185	American Home Products (Wyeth-Ayerst)	Contraception	Ethinyl estradiol and levonorgestrel
Noroxin	156	Merck (MS&D)	Infection	Norfloxacin
Ogen	162	Abbott	Menopause symptoms	Estropipate
Ortho-novum 1/35-21	189	Johnson & Johnson (Ortho Pharm)	Contraception	Ethinyl estradiol and norethindrone
Ortho-novum 1/35-28	62	Johnson & Johnson (Ortho Pharm)	Contraception	Ethinyl estradiol and norethindrone
Ortho-novum 7/7/7-21	153	Johnson & Johnson (Ortho Pharm)	Contraception	Ethinyl estradiol and norethindrone
Ortho-novum 7/7/7-28	22	Johnson & Johnson (Ortho Pharm)	Contraception	Ethinyl estradiol and norethindrone
Orudis	95	American Home Products (Wyeth-Ayerst)	Arthritis; pain	Ketoprofen
Pamelor	52	Sandoz	Depression	Nortriptyline HCl
PCE 333	142	Abbott	Infection	Erythromycin base
PCE 500	117	Abbott	Infection	Erythromycin base
Penicillin VK	76	Mylan	Infection	Penicillin V potassium
Penicillin VK	164	Warner-Lambert (Warner Chilcott)	Infection	Penicillin V potassium
Pen-Vee K	75	American Home Products (Wyeth-Ayerst)	Infection	Penicillin V potassium
Pepcid	49	Merck (MS&D)	Ulcers	Famotidine

Drug	Rank	Manufacturer	Purpose	Chemical or Brand Name
Percocet	136	Du Pont Merck Pharmaceutical	Pain	Oxycodone and acetaminophen
Peridex	170	Procter & Gamble	Dental infection	Chlorhexidine
Persantine	145	Boehringer Ingelheim	Blood clots	Dipyridamole
Phenergan	149	American Home Products (Wyeth-Ayerst)	Cough	Promethazine
Polymox	46	Bristol-Myers Squibb (Apothecon)	Infection	Amoxicillin trihydrate
Prednisone*	176	Rugby Labs	Inflammation	Generic version of Deltasone
Premarin	2	American Home Products (Wyeth-Ayerst)	Menopause, osteoporosis	Conjugated estrogen
Prilosec	152	Merck (MS&D)	Ulcers	Omeprazole
Prinivil	59	Merck (MS&D)	Cardiovascular disease	Lisinopril
Procardia	96	Pfizer	Cardiovascular disease	Nifedipine
Procardia XL	10	Pfizer	Cardiovascular disease	Nifedipine
Propacet 100	92	Lemmon Company	Arthritis; pain	Propoxyphene napsylate and acetaminophen
Propine	191	Allergan	Glaucoma	Dipivetrin HCl
Propoxyphene napsylate and acetaminophen*	64	Mylan	Arthritis; pain	Generic version of Darvocet-N
Propoxyphene napsylate and acetaminophen*	188	Rugby Labs	Arthritis; pain	Generic version of Darvocet-N
Propranolol*	199	Lederle	Cardiovascular disease, migraine	Generic version of Inderal
Proventil aerosol	20	Schering-Plough (Schering)	Asthma	Albuterol
Proventil nebulizer	147	Schering-Plough	Asthma	Albuterol
Proventil tabs	128	Schering-Plough	Asthma	Albuterol
Provera	28	Upjohn	Abnormal uterine bleeding	Medroxyprogesterone
Prozac	19	Eli Lilly (Dista)	Depression	Fluoxetine HCl
Reglan	187	American Home Products (Wyeth-Ayerst)	Digestion problems	Metoclopramide
Restoril	160	Sandoz	Insomnia	Temazepam
Retin-A	123	Johnson & Johnson (Ortho Derm)	Acne	Trentinoin
Rogaine	179	Upjohn	Hair loss	Minoxidil
Seldane	9	Marion Merrell Dow	Allergy	Terfenadine
Sinemet	127	Du Pont Merck Pharmaceutical	Parkinson's disease	Carbidopa and levodopa
Slo-Bid	99	Rhône-Poulenc Rorer	Asthma	Theophylline
Slow-K	97	Ciba-Geigy (Summit)	Potassium deficiency	Potassium chloride in wax
Sumycin	169	Bristol-Myers Squibb (Apothecon)	Infection	Tetracycline
Suprax	112	Lederle	Infection	Cefixime
Synthroid	6	Boots Pharmaceuticals	Thyroid deficiency	Levothyroxine sodium
Tagamet	15	SmithKline Beecham	Ulcers	Cimetidine
Tavist D	71	Sandoz	Decongestant	Phenylpropanolamine and clemastine fumarate
Tegretol	73	Ciba-Geigy (Basel)	Epilepsy	Carbamazepine
Tenex	143	American Home Products (Robins)	Cardiovascular disease	Guanfacine HCl
Tenoretic	141	ICI Americas	Cardiovascular disease	Atenolol and chlorthalidone
Tenormin	11	ICI Americas	Cardiovascular disease	Atenolol
Terazol 7	106	Johnson & Johnson (Ortho Pharm)	Infection	Terconazole
Theo-Dur	35	Schering-Plough (Key)	Asthma	Theophylline
Thyroid	126	Forest Laboratories	Thyroid deficiency	Thyroid desiccated
Timoptic	51	Merck (MS&D)	Glaucoma	Timolol maleate
Tobrex	190	Alcon	Infection	Tobramycin
Transderm-Nitro	94	Ciba-Geigy (Summit)	Chest pains	Nitroglycerine
Trental	65	Hoechst-Roussel	Blood thinner	Pentoxifylline
Triamterene and hydrochlorthiazide*	61	Rugby Labs	Cardiovascular disease	Generic version of Dyazide
Tri-levlen 28	104	Berlex	Contraception	Levonorgestrel and ethinyl estradiol
Trimethoprim and sulfamethoxazole*	134	Biocraft	Infection	Generic version of Bactrim and Septra
Trimethoprim and sulfamethoxazole*	155	Rugby Labs	Infection	Generic version of Bactrim and Septra
Trimethoprim and sulfamethoxazole*	165	Mutual Pharmaceuticals	Infection	Generic version of Bactrim and Septra
Trimox	31	Bristol-Myers Squibb (Apothecon)	Infection	Amoxicillin trihydrate

Drug	Rank	Manufacturer	Purpose	Chemical or Brand Name
Triphasil-28	40	American Home Products (Wyeth-Ayerst)	Contraception	Levonorgestrel and ethinyl estradiol
Tylenol with Codeine	36	Johnson & Johnson (McNeil Pharm)	Pain	Codeine phosphate and acetaminophen
Valium	60	Roche Laboratories	Anxiety	Diazepam
Vancenase-AQ	102	Schering-Plough	Asthma	Beclomethasone dipropionate
Vanceril	168	Schering-Plough	Asthma	Beclomethasone dipropionate
Vaseretic	193	Merck (MS&D)	Cardiovascular disease	Enalapril maleate and hydrochlorothiazide
Vasotec	8	Merck (MS&D)	Cardiovascular disease	Enalapril
Veetids	93	Bristol-Myers Squibb (Apothecon)	Infection	Penicillin V potassium
Ventolin aerosol	25	Glaxo (Allen & Hanburys)	Asthma	Albuterol
Ventolin syrup	103	Glaxo (Allen & Hanburys)	Asthma	Albuterol
Verelan	184	Lederle	Cardiovascular disease	Verapamil HCl
Vicodin	72	Knoll	Pain	Hydrocodone and acetaminophen
Vicodin ES	118	Knoll	Pain	Hydrocodone and acetaminophen
Voltaren	30	Ciba-Geigy (Geigy)	Arthritis; pain	Diclofenac
Wymox	119	American Home Products (Wyeth-Ayerst)	Infection	Amoxicillin trihydrate
Xanax	5	Upjohn	Anxiety	Alprazolam
Zantac	3	Glaxo	Ulcers	Ranitidine
Zestril	48	ICI Americas (Stuart)	Cardiovascular disease	Lisinopril
Zovirax capsules	79	Burroughs Wellcome	Viral infection	Acyclovir
Zovirax ointment	195	Burroughs Wellcome	Viral infection	Acyclovir